Anatomy of Movement
EXERCISES

Originally published as *Anatomie pour le mouvement, tome 2: bases d'exercices,* Editions Desiris (France), 1990. Revised in 1992.

English language edition © 1996 by Eastland Press, Incorporated
P.O. Box 99749, Seattle, WA 98199 USA
All rights reserved.

Library of Congress Card Number: 94-61964
International Standard Book Number: 0-939616-22-X
Printed in the United States of America

4 6 8 10 9 7 5

English language edition translated by Nicole Commarmond,
edited by Stephen Anderson, Ph.D.

Book design by Gary Niemeier
Typesetting by Gordon Frazier

Our thanks to the models
for the photographs in this book:

the students of
Danse-Creation (Lille, France)
Studio l'Eix (Palafrugell, Spain)

and in particular,

Sylvie Battault
Cathy Carbonne
Marie-Helene Paradowski
Bernard Coignard

Table of Contents

Preface

This book is the natural sequel to *Anatomy of Movement*, referred to hereafter as *AOM*.

Who is our intended audience?

- Primarily people who teach some form of physical exercise (especially classes for beginners, children, or "amateurs") and need some guidelines in choosing specific exercises or progressions.

- Students or practitioners of physical disciplines such as dance, martial arts, yoga, or sports.

- Therapists who use exercise as part of their treatment program.

What does this book offer?

Working from the anatomical framework and point of view introduced in *AOM*, this book describes a comprehensive series of exercises selected for both efficiency and harmlessness. Some work the whole body, while others focus on particular regions.

These exercises prepare the body to respond well to the demands of specified movements. They can be used as a basis for teaching or learning other more specialized or complex exercises in various physical disciplines. Thus, they provide a supporting or enriching "tool" for these other disciplines.

Organization

After an introductory chapter, there are a series of chapters, each representing a region of the body. The sequence of regions is the same as in *AOM*: trunk, shoulder, elbow/forearm, wrist/hand, hip, knee, and ankle/foot. The anatomical concepts explained in *AOM* provide the basis for the descriptions in this volume as well, so we strongly recommend that the reader already be familiar with *AOM*, or have it available for reference.

For each region we provide or describe:

- an introduction and special comments
- characteristic movements
- basis for flexibility: sources of stiffness or laxity and how to detect, prevent, or overcome them
- muscles or muscle groups, and ways to strengthen specific muscles
- coordination of movements in the region.

From time to time we synthesize or summarize preceding material, or point out common themes.

For each region, we provide many "practice pages" which include:

- test and assessment exercises
- basic exercises (marked with asterisk) appropriate for almost any class
- special exercises that can be done less frequently during class
- exercises that should be done at home, since there is usually not enough time in class (e.g., fine mobilization exercises of the foot).

Obviously, no one can expect to do all the exercises shown in this book in one session. They must be spread over a period of several months or years.

Although the exercises are shown in their entirety, they should be taught in a gradual, sequential manner before the teacher requests execution of the complete exercise.

In the practice pages, some exercises are specifically designed for children or older adults, and are indicated as such.

CHAPTER ONE

Introduction

Exercises described in the practice pages are categorized according to purpose:

- **increase flexibility**
- **strengthen muscles**
- **coordinate movement.**

These three goals are sometimes confused. A ballet teacher may suggest a series of pliés "to develop flexibility in the lower limbs." However, if flexibility is the goal, there are alternative exercises much more efficient than the plié. During pliés, the hip joint does not attain maximum range of motion (ROM), and certain hip and knee muscles are not elongated at all. In fact, the plié serves a different purpose: to develop, through habitual repetition, more refined coordination of a series of small movements found in all jumps, and thereby help protect the joints from stress injury.

In teaching or practicing the exercises in this book, the reader should clearly distinguish among these three goals.

Exercises to warm up and increase flexibility

The purpose of these exercises is to preserve good ROM, or attain greater ROM. Flexibility varies greatly from person to person depending on many factors such as age, weight, lifestyle, arthritis, and prior injuries to joints. Within an individual, flexibility varies among different joints or even between the same joint on opposite sides of the body.

Flexibility or lack of flexibility (stiffness) at joints is determined by three components: bones, connective tissues, and surrounding muscles.

Bones permit or restrict movements according to the shape of the bones and their articular facets. For example, the shape of the lumbar vertebrae restricts rotation (see *AOM*, p. 50).

Connective tissues include discs or cartilage within the joint, and capsules and ligaments outside the joint. Stiffness attributable to connective tissue structures is rare in children, moderately common in adults, and very common in older adults. We will present exercises which

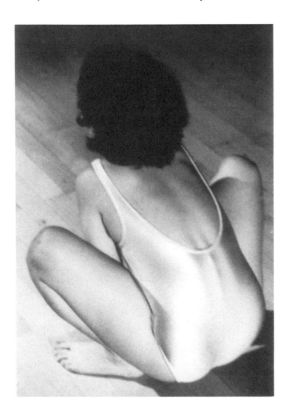

specifically improve "sweeping" of cartilages by synovial fluid, which are helpful for older adults. Joint capsules and ligaments allow the characteristic movement of the joint while preventing the bones from being displaced from their proper positions. Their elasticity is quite limited. If capsules or ligaments are overstretched, they do not readily return to their original length. They are well supplied with sensitive nerves which send a signal to the brain when they are stretched. If ligaments are overstretched, these "stretch receptors" no longer relay accurate information to the brain, and the risk of sprain is increased. This is particularly true for certain ligaments of the feet, knees, and spine, which should therefore not be overstretched during warm–up exercises.

On the other hand, the anterior ligaments of the hip and certain spinal ligaments (different from those mentioned above) are often "folded" on themselves, and exercises designed to "unfold" them will help them recover their proper length.

In contrast to connective tissues, the **muscles** associated with a joint are both contractile and elastic. Muscles can act as brakes in certain movements, either because their connective tissue covering (fascia or aponeurosis) is tight, or because their fibers exhibit tonus (chronic contraction) and resist lengthening. Flexibility exercises are typically designed to stretch the fascia and/or fibers of muscles. To stretch a monoarticular muscle (one that crosses only one joint), we need to perform a movement opposite to its action. To stretch a polyarticular muscle, we need to perform an exercise which involves all the joints crossed by the muscle.

As an example, let's consider stretching of the rectus femoris (see *AOM*, pp. 217–19).

1. Simple stretching

The body is placed in a position which increases the distance between the origin and insertion of the muscle, but not so far as to create a burning or tearing sensation. Simply holding this position will tend to lengthen the muscle. However, it is important that the movement to attain the position be done slowly, since a quick movement may provoke a shortening reflex of the muscle.

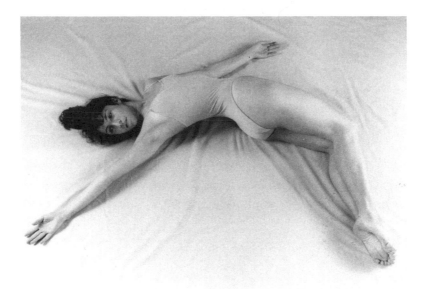

2. Muscular release

This method increases length of a muscle without risk of tearing the fibers or fascia. A muscle never relaxes completely during ordinary movements. In order to attain the maximal muscular relaxation ("release") possible, it is essential that the joint involved not be in any need of support, nor risk of dislocation. For example, if the arm is freely dangling in space, the shoulder muscles will be in tonic contraction because of the need to support the shoulder joint. Likewise, if the shoulder joint is taken into a movement at the limit of ROM, there will be muscular contraction to avoid dislocation.

Therefore, to achieve muscular release, the joint should be completely supported and nowhere near the limit of ROM. In the case of the rectus femoris, start with the foot held in the hand, without trying to stretch the muscle further through traction of the foot (see *AOM*, p. 219). Wait awhile before stretching further through involvement of the pelvis or foot.

3. Contraction/relaxation

This method utilizes the latency period that follows muscular contraction to stretch the muscle. In the rectus femoris example, start with the muscle in a position just before stretching. Then try to extend the knee (the foot pushes the hand; the rectus femoris contracts). Maintain this intense contraction for a few seconds, then release the muscle. Elongation is facilitated if you do not approach the limit of ROM, nor stretch too quickly.

Strengthening exercises

The goal of these exercises is to increase the strength of contraction of specific muscles, to facilitate specific actions in a physical discipline. Beyond early childhood (4–5 years), the life style of the typical person in today's society does not provide for sufficient growth or maintenance of muscular strength. In many adults, the muscles actually tend to become weaker over time. A well-designed exercise program can maintain or increase muscular strength. You should be aware of some important principles:

- For a muscle to increase in strength or size, it must be put in sustained or repeated maximal contraction, far beyond what is encountered in normal daily activities.
- Between contractions, the muscle needs adequate time to relax. This is necessary for the quality of the contraction that will follow.
- During exercise, the body must receive sufficient oxygen and expel carbon dioxide. The exercise room must be well-ventilated during and between sessions. You should breathe deeply before, during, and after the exercise. In this way you will avoid cramps and aching muscles.

Static contraction

This involves no visible bodily movement. Muscular contraction serves simply to maintain a certain posture. Example: "freezing" during a movement without returning to resting position — lifting the leg and keeping it raised.

Advantages:
- Exercises the muscle without articular movement, and therefore without fatigue of the cartilage.
- Allows one to work on very precise placements.

Disadvantages:
- Students who are looking for a lot of activity may feel they "aren't doing anything."
- Muscular fatigue may set in if intense static contraction is held for longer than seven seconds.

Dynamic contraction

Muscular contraction produces visible bodily movement. Example: contraction of the deltoid elevates the arm, or acts as a brake as the arm is slowly lowered from the elevated position.

Advantages:
- Associated with movement, which is pleasing to students.
- Requires less relaxation time because contraction of a particular muscle will typically alternate with that of its opposing muscle.

Disadvantages:
- Does not permit as much precision as static contraction.
- Causes friction of cartilage or bone in the joint.

Most muscular strengthening exercises in this book can be performed in either static or dynamic mode.

Discussion of cardiovascular and other physiological aspects of these exercises, and descriptions of breathing exercises (particularly diaphragmatic breathing), are outside the scope of this book, but can readily be found elsewhere by the interested reader.

Coordination exercises

How do these differ from muscle strengthening exercises?

Movement coordination implies an increase not of the quantitative strength of a muscle, but of its involvement in successive movements that make up complex actions. We can increase strength in the finger muscles by squeezing a rubber ball. However, this will be of little help in learning how to play the piano or type on a computer keyboard. Learning to coordinate finger movements in these complex actions will require a different type of exercise.

Any physical discipline requires specialized forms of complex coordinated movements (posting in horseback riding, serving in tennis, pirouettes in dance). However, there are more fundamental coordination exercises which are useful for all these specialized movements. The fundamental exercises are described in this book.

The practice pages in this book introduce some general tests and exercises falling in the three categories described above (flexibility, strength, coordination). They are usually separated, but may be combined in some cases (e.g., chapter on the foot) to avoid excessive length or repetition. Also, some exercises may involve two or even all three of these elements.

CHAPTER TWO

The Trunk & Neck

....

The trunk, neck, and head comprise the central (median) part of the body. The paired shoulder and pelvic girdles, and the limbs, are attached to the trunk. We will follow the traditional division of the posterior bony structure of the trunk (the vertebral column or spine) into **lumbar**, **thoracic**, and **cervical** regions. Remember that because of the number of vertebrae and the joints between them, the spine is extremely mobile (see *AOM*, chapter 2).

The hollow spaces (foramina) of the vertebrae line up to form the vertebral canal, which surrounds and protects the spinal cord. Spinal nerves branch off the spinal cord and exit between vertebrae to carry nerve signals to and from all the muscles and organs of the body.

Good mobility and tone of the muscles supporting the vertebral column are important throughout life, and particularly in the later years.

Movements

Because of the mobility of the spine, the trunk can move easily in all three dimensions.

Movements in the sagittal plane
are called **flexion** . . .

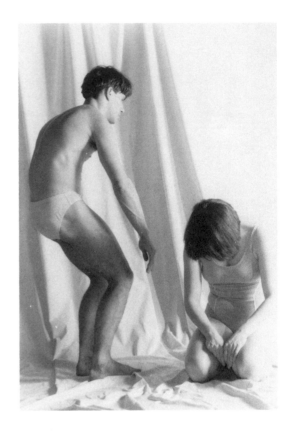

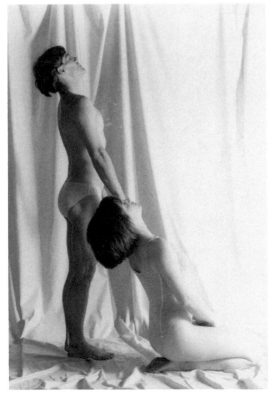

. . . and **extension**.

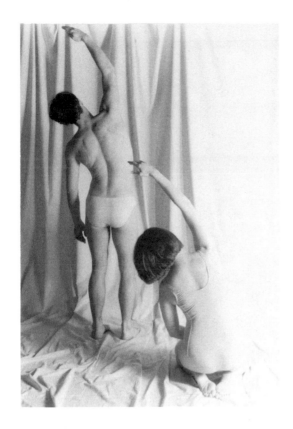

Movements in the frontal (coronal) plane are called **lateral flexion** or **side-bending**.

Movements in the transverse (horizontal) plane are called **rotation**.

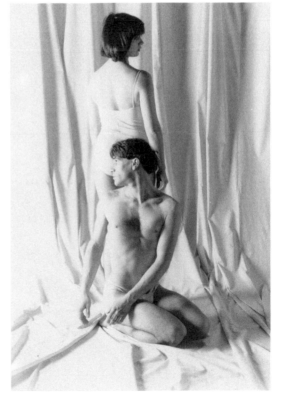

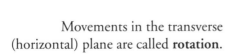

ROM of these movements is different at every vertebral level. The spine is not a snake-like structure with mobilities evenly distributed along its entire length. Some areas are more specialized for flexion, others for rotation, extension, or side-bending. Some areas are much more mobile than others.

Vertebral structure

A brief review of anatomy (see *AOM*, pp. 32–3).

The anterior part of the vertebra is the massive **body**, designed to bear weight. The **posterior arch** and its foramen enclose the nerve structures: the spinal cord (with its meninges), and the spinal nerves that exit at each level.

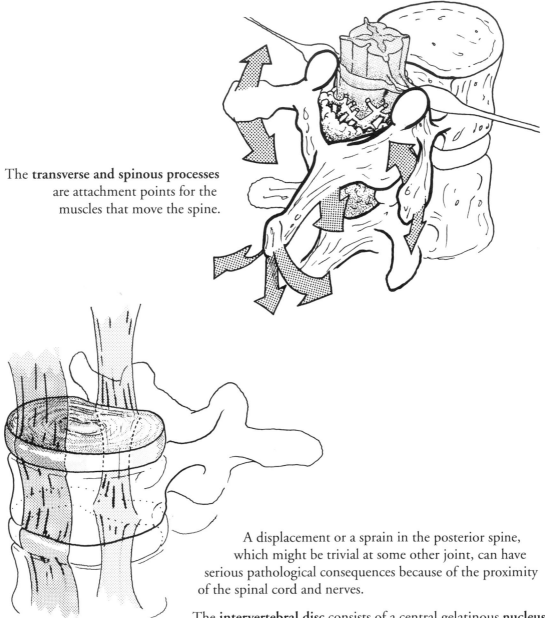

The **transverse and spinous processes** are attachment points for the muscles that move the spine.

A displacement or a sprain in the posterior spine, which might be trivial at some other joint, can have serious pathological consequences because of the proximity of the spinal cord and nerves.

The **intervertebral disc** consists of a central gelatinous **nucleus pulposus** and a peripheral fibrocartilage **annulus fibrosus**, concentrically layered around the nucleus. The disc acts as a shock absorber, and can alter its shape. The discs are attached to the vertebral bodies by thin layers of cartilage, and are collectively held in place by the **posterior and anterior longitudinal ligaments**, which adhere to the discs and vertebral bodies respectively (see *AOM*, pp. 33–4).

Behavior of the weight-bearing disc

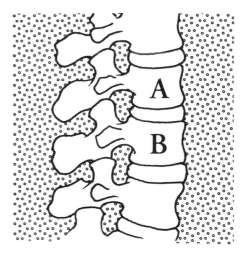

Consider a disc situated between two adjacent vertebral bodies, which we will term A (above) and B (below).

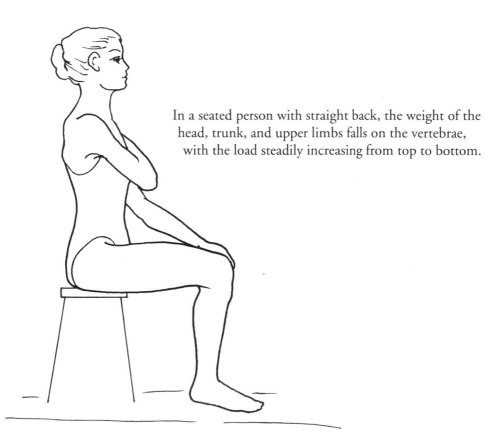

In a seated person with straight back, the weight of the head, trunk, and upper limbs falls on the vertebrae, with the load steadily increasing from top to bottom.

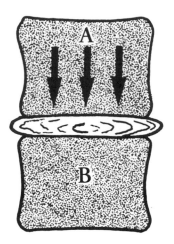

If the nucleus were absent, the load on the disc would produce a compression of the fibers in the annulus.

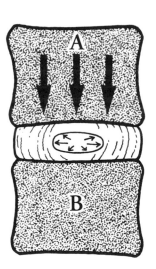

However, the nucleus tends to transmit or distribute the pressure in all directions. The fibers of the annulus are put under tension, and this reduces their compression.

As long as the spine remains straight and vertically aligned (with its normal curves), the load is evenly distributed through each disc at each level, which is an ideal shock-absorbing condition. In this way, the disc can bear heavy loads without damage. In some cultures, people are accustomed to carrying heavy objects on their heads throughout much of their lives and do not suffer back problems.

Consequences of forward bending the spine

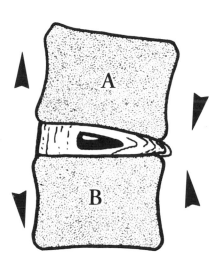

Consider now an "unevenly distributed" load which compresses the disc anteriorly and stretches it posteriorly.

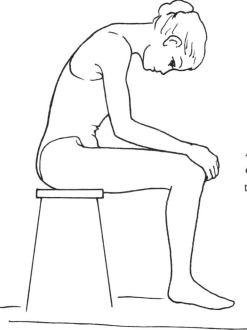

At the level of the L5/S1 junction, the weight of the upper body is not falling vertically on the disc, but considerably anterior to it.

This distance magnifies the strain on the disc, just as your strength can be magnified by using a lever. The strain is further magnified if the subject's arms in this example are held out in front of the body, and especially if they are holding some extra weight. The kinetic energy imparted by movement (e.g., leaping forward) can further magnify the strain.

In this situation, we would like the spinal muscles to partially counteract the strain of compression on the anterior disc and stretching on the posterior disc. Strong contraction of posterior muscles would limit the posterior stretching of the disc.

Unfortunately, these muscles are usually not exercised sufficiently. Many people let their spines "collapse" for hours on end by slouching on soft couches, office chairs, or car seats, with the unintentional effect of fatiguing the intervertebral discs.

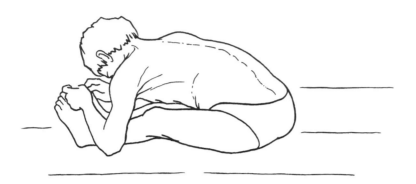

Furthermore, various forward-bending "exercises" intended to make the spine more supple aggravate the type of disc strain described above.

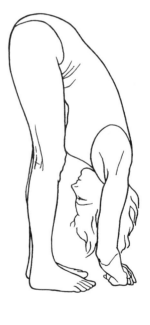

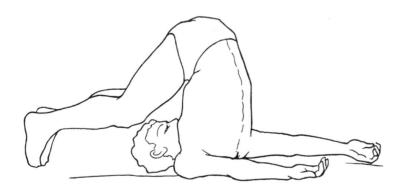

What happens to a disc if chronically aggravated in these ways?
- It may gradually degenerate and dry up.
- Cracks may appear which make the annulus less watertight.
- Fluid from the nucleus may escape through the annulus via the cracks.

Let's look now at the consequences of forward bending on the ligaments, taking two lumbar vertebrae as an example.

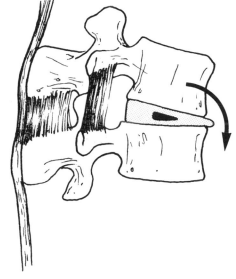

The first ligament to be put under tension is the supraspinous ligament, followed by the interspinous ligament and those between the transverse processes.

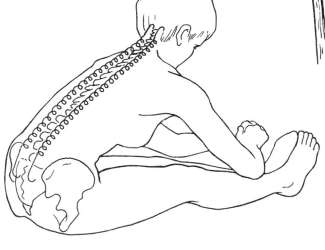

In reality, these ligaments are not strong enough to resist extreme forward bending, or bending which is maintained for a long time. Contraction of posterior spinal muscles is essential to counteract the strain.

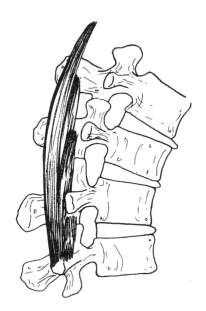

An example is the multifidus spinae shown here (see also *AOM*, pp. 64–5).

If contraction of these muscles is "deprogrammed" by chronic slouching or other causes, the ligaments and discs will become fatigued, and the person may eventually experience diffuse and chronic lumbar backache, called "**lumbago**." The distended ligaments will progressively weaken and cease to inform the brain of their strained condition.

In this situation, a sudden, "loaded" forward-bending movement can overstretch the posterior longitudinal ligament.

This is serious because of the strategic location of the ligament inside the spinal canal, anterior to the spinal cord. There is no "free space" here; the spinal cord, meninges, and cerebrospinal fluid fill the spinal canal. Edema (swelling) resulting from overstretching of the ligament will cause immediate and acute pain.

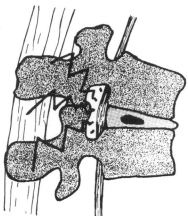

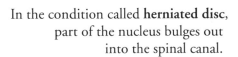

This edema may also compress the nerve roots where they exit from the canal. The most common case is compression of the **sciatic nerves**, which exit from intervertebral foramina L4/L5, L5/S1, and the first three sacral foramina.

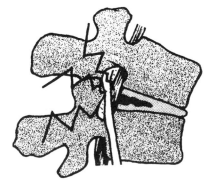

In the condition called **herniated disc**, part of the nucleus bulges out into the spinal canal.

The likelihood or severity of all these pathological phenomena is increased when weight, traction, or abrupt movement is added to the forward bending.

We hope you now appreciate how flexing exercises intended to make the spine more "supple" may actually seriously weaken or damage the lumbar spine.

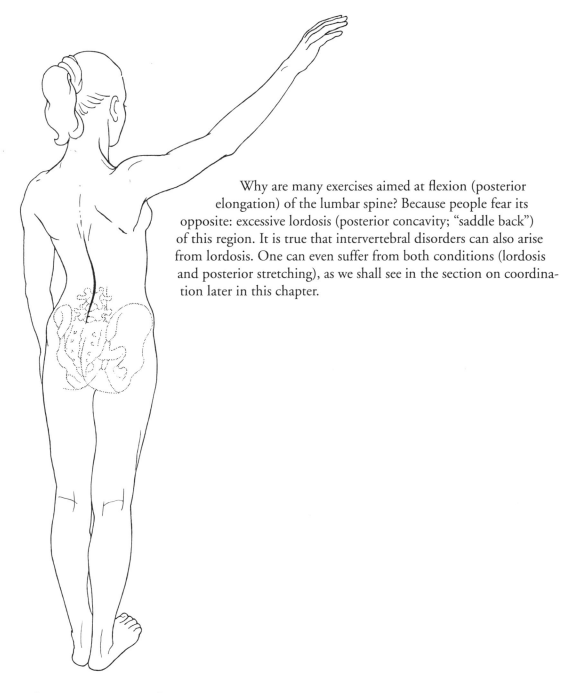

Why are many exercises aimed at flexion (posterior elongation) of the lumbar spine? Because people fear its opposite: excessive lordosis (posterior concavity; "saddle back") of this region. It is true that intervertebral disorders can also arise from lordosis. One can even suffer from both conditions (lordosis and posterior stretching), as we shall see in the section on coordination later in this chapter.

A few important principles:
- The vertebral discs must be allowed some resting time. This means that the discs are vertically aligned and without any peripheral loading.
- A limbering exercise, if it affects a curvature of the spine, should never involve any loading.
- A spine flexibility exercise can be harmful if improperly done (especially for a beginner or a very "stiff" individual) because of the location and function of the spinal cord.
- Practitioners or students of physical disciplines should build up strength in the muscles supporting the trunk, particularly the deep muscles, and coordinate the actions of these muscles in such a way that they distribute loads evenly on the vertebral discs.

Flexibility of the spine

Flexibility or suppleness of the spine is important for and characteristic of children. Obviously, we do not want to lose flexibility. However, you should understand that, in adults, backaches generally occur not in stiff areas, but in poorly managed mobile areas. *You should not practice or teach exercises aimed at "limbering" the spine unless other exercises for maintaining good support of the spine are taught first.* Normal flexibility is good, but excessive mobility is not.

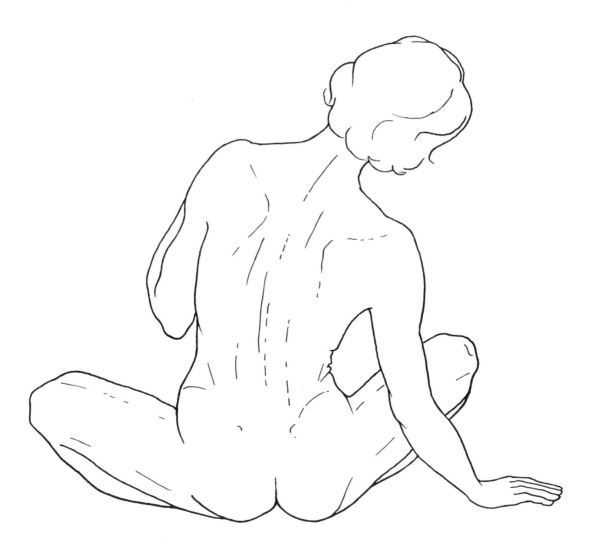

Although many of our exercises are aimed at increasing ROM (e.g., greater degree of extension, lateral flexion), we always prefer situations where the vertebrae are *not loaded*.

Why?

Because the limit of ROM is reached using movements that *put the spine in a precariously balanced situation*. There is no need to add further strain by imposing a load. In classroom exercises focused on flexibility of the spine, we choose movements where the load on the vertebrae is minimal, and concentrate on getting as far as possible in completing the movement.

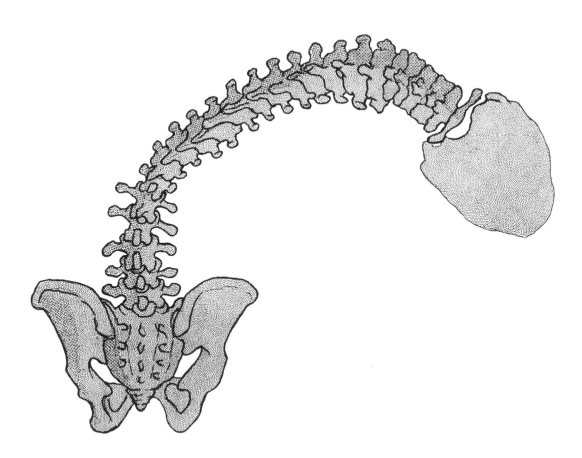

Mobility of the spine varies by region

During stretching exercises, the most mobile regions may be overly solicited.

Areas of hypermobility are found in hinge-like transitional situations, where we pass from one type of vertebra to another.

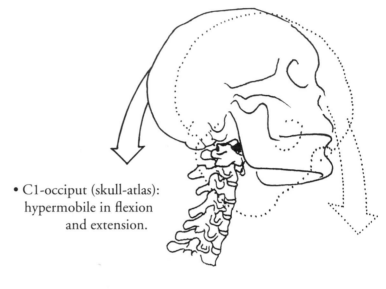

• C1-occiput (skull-atlas): hypermobile in flexion and extension.

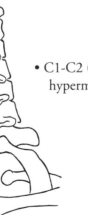

• C1-C2 (atlas-axis): hypermobile in rotation.

• C7-T1: hypermobile in flexion. This is a transition from a region of limited flexion (thoracic spine) to a region of great flexion (cervical spine).

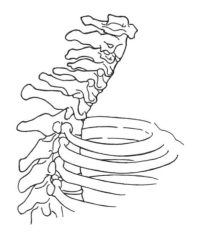

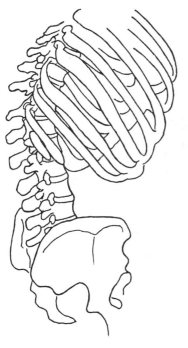

• T12-L1:
hypermobile
in flexion,

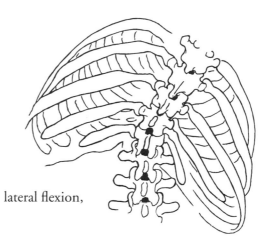

lateral flexion,

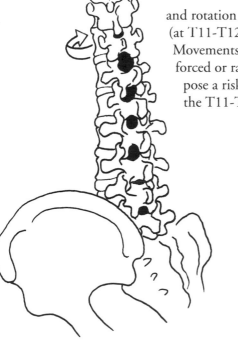

and rotation
(at T11-T12).
Movements involving
forced or rapid rotation
pose a risk of injuring
the T11-T12 disc.

• L5-S1: hypermobile
in extension. This is the
joint subject to strain
when arching the back.

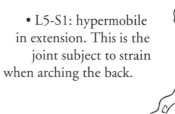

Between these hinge areas, characteristic mobilities are also observed:

• The cervical region is hypermobile in most directions. We will see that stiffness of the neck or restriction of movements here is often due to muscles rather than joints.

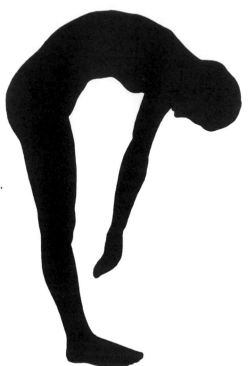

• Although the thoracic region has a characteristic posterior convexity (kyphosis), flexion of the upper thoracic spine is restricted by the presence of the ribs and sternum.

• The lumbar region has a tendency toward extension.

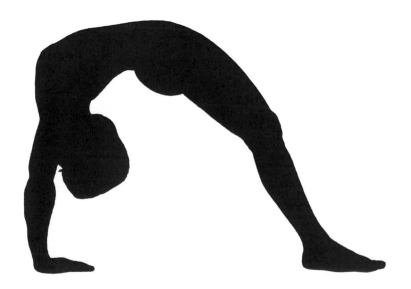

Movements that occur in areas of extreme mobility should be performed carefully, or with deliberately limited range. For example:

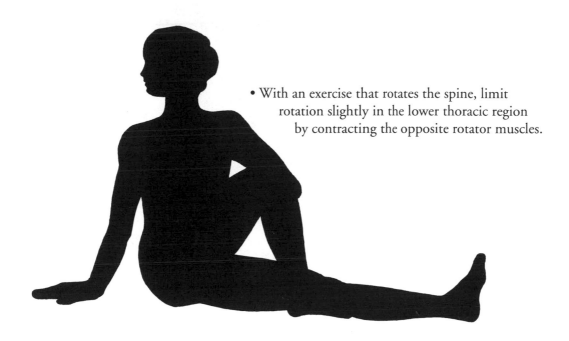

- With an exercise that rotates the spine, limit rotation slightly in the lower thoracic region by contracting the opposite rotator muscles.

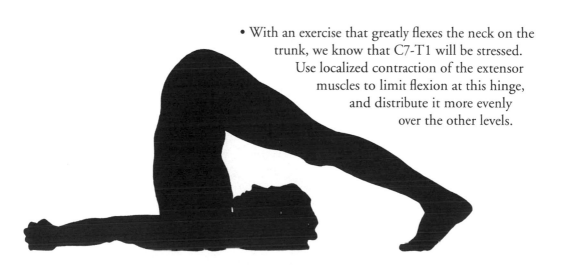

- With an exercise that greatly flexes the neck on the trunk, we know that C7-T1 will be stressed. Use localized contraction of the extensor muscles to limit flexion at this hinge, and distribute it more evenly over the other levels.

We also need to make the spine more supple *longitudinally*, as if stretching it from the occiput to the sacrum.

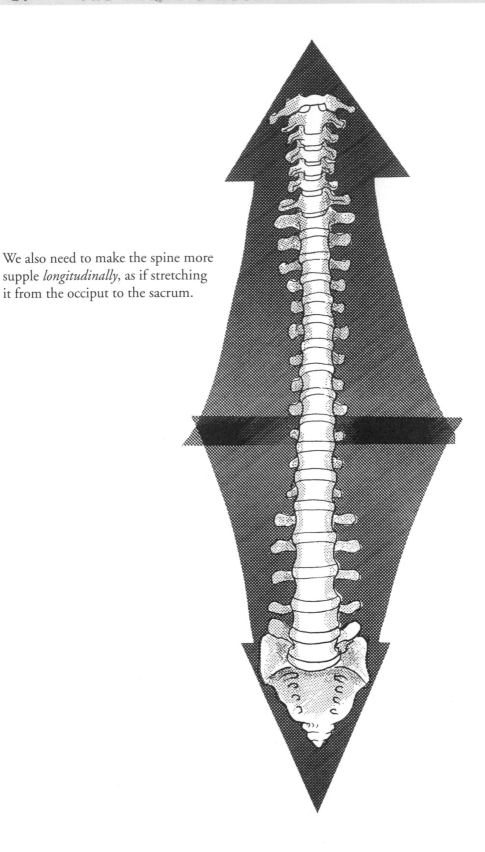

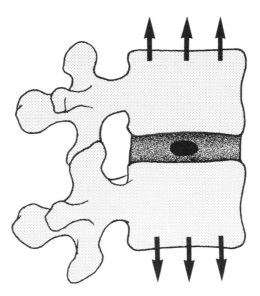

When the spine is aligned and not loaded ("off-load"), especially if a slight longitudinal traction is added, the intervertebral discs are decompressed and their nuclei recover the normal, central position. This is the opposite of what happens when the spine is loaded.

Different spinal regions respond differently to longitudinal stretching. Simple head-sacrum traction exercises stretch mainly weak points such as C4 and T12-L1. Therefore, we present two types of longitudinal stretching exercises: one in which the spine is stretched one region at a time (precise but time-consuming), and a more general type (quicker and easier but not as precise).

Muscles of the trunk

The deep vs. superficial muscles of the trunk are easy to distinguish in terms of size and function as well as location.

The **deep muscles** typically form numerous small bundles which run from one vertebra to the next, from one vertebra to the next two or three, or from the vertebrae to the ribs. They are capable of acting very precisely to maintain or adjust the alignment of vertebrae with respect to each other. On the other hand, because they are small and located very close to the bones they move, they have little leverage and exert little force. They are not responsible for large-scale or powerful movements, but rather work constantly to maintain or recover proper stacking of the vertebrae. For instance, we hold our head and spine in an upright position while standing or sitting, without thinking about it, thanks to the constant activity and coordination of deep muscles.

The **superficial muscles** are located closer to the skin. They are much more massive and longer than the deep muscles, and span greater distances. They have greater leverage and force, but less precision than the deep muscles. They are responsible for large ROM actions such as extension or sidebending of the spine or head. Their action is intermittent and powerful.

Deep spinal muscles (anterior)

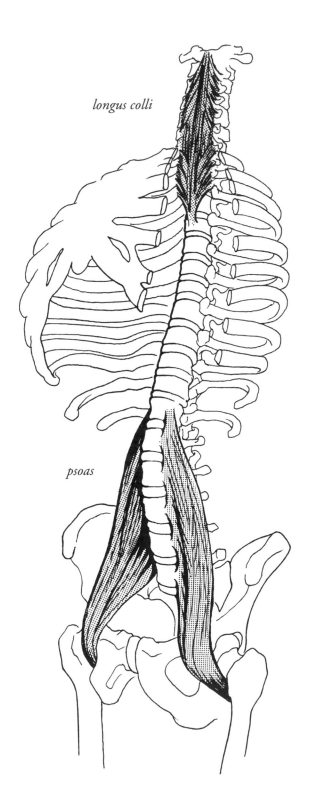

longus colli

psoas

Deep spinal muscles (posterior)

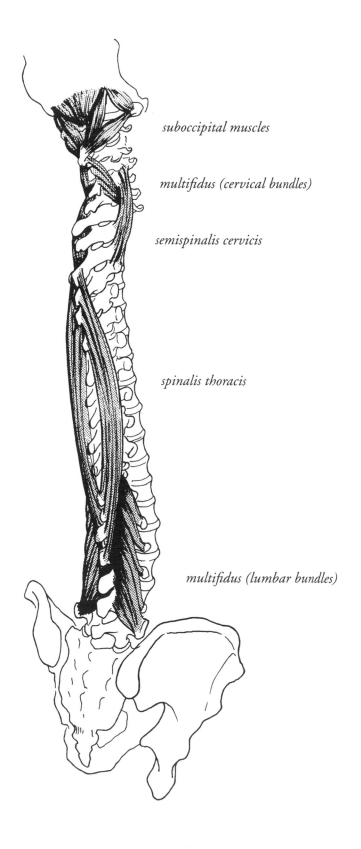

suboccipital muscles

multifidus (cervical bundles)

semispinalis cervicis

spinalis thoracis

multifidus (lumbar bundles)

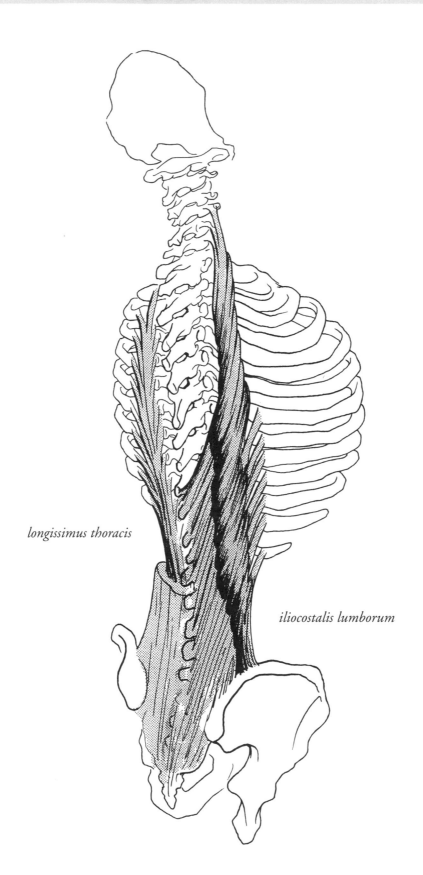

longissimus thoracis

iliocostalis lumborum

Superficial spinal muscles (anterior)

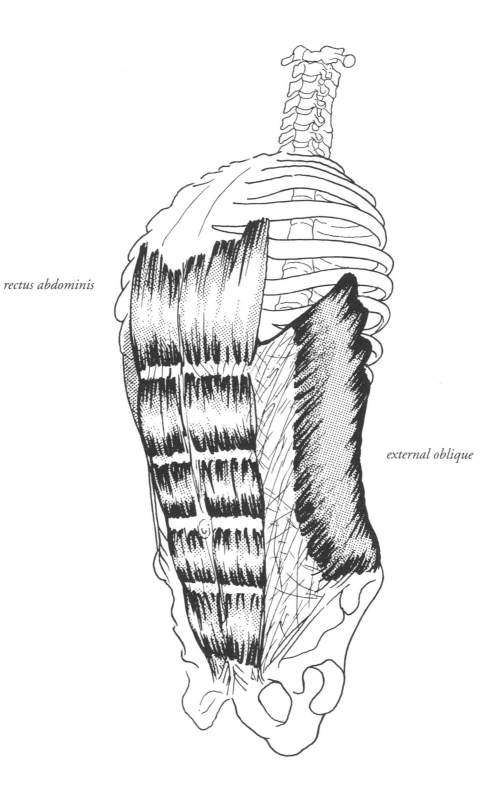

rectus abdominis

external oblique

Superficial spinal muscles (posterior)

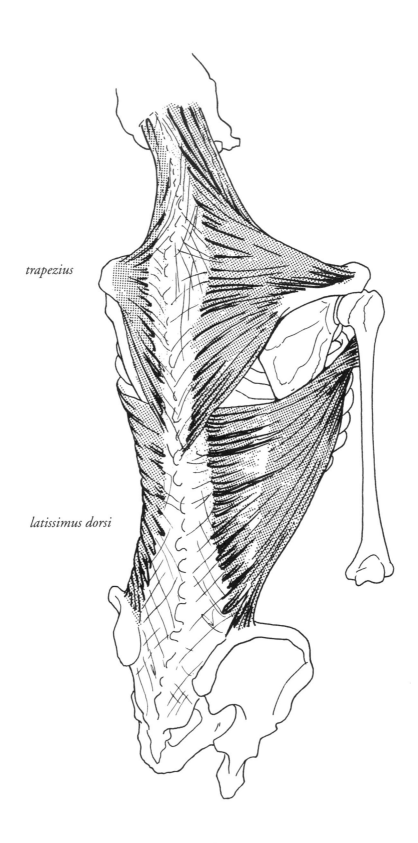

trapezius

latissimus dorsi

Functional and practical considerations

The deep muscles of the trunk help us maintain an erect or upright posture even when the body's center of gravity is altered, e.g., when we raise one arm or leg, or tilt the head. These muscles are small and "close to the bone." When you practice exercises directed at them, e.g., vertical alignment of the spine, expect a sensation of very slight muscular contraction. With a vertically erect trunk, the superficial muscles are used for actions of large ROM and brief duration, e.g., leaning forward or arching the back.

You should always be aware of the distinction between deep vs. superficial muscles, and their functions, and practice or teach exercises focused on both groups (separately or together). This is important in today's world because people are suffering from back problems at a progressively younger age. In people who spend years slouching on chairs, the deep spinal muscles become "deprogrammed," and assuming an erect posture requires conscious effort. The superficial muscles may even be called upon to take over the work of the deep muscles, which is inappropriate because they are not designed to be postural muscles, nor to contract for sustained periods of time. In this situation, the superficial muscles may go into spasm or generate sensations of diffuse pain. The person, seeking a more comfortable position, will look for a soft armchair or a seat with a back to lean on, or will simply let his/her back "collapse." These actions will provide some relief to the muscles, but at the expense of excessive loading of the intervertebral discs, which we obviously wish to avoid.

How can the deep muscles be "awakened" to assume their proper function? Either by tactile stimulation, or by specific exercises such as those shown in the practice section.

For the strength exercises of the deep as well as superficial spinal muscles, we are not looking to increase ROM (in contrast to the flexibility exercises), but to stimulate and contract as many muscles and muscle fibers as possible.

For a given spinal region, there is a relatively convex side and a concave side; for example, the lumbar spine is convex anteriorly and concave posteriorly. For bending exercises, our general rule is to elongate (enlarge) the concave side, i.e., reduce the degree of concavity. However, no muscles located within the concave side can accomplish this; such muscles, by contracting, can only accentuate the concavity.

The muscles able to reduce the concavity are those located on the convex side. It is their braking action which limits ROM and prevents compression on the concave side. In a beginners' class of older adults, we avoid any loaded bending whatsoever until the students develop stronger muscles. Beyond a certain age, the discs lose some of their resistance to pressure. We recommend starting out with movements which bend the spine as a whole from the hips, thereby strengthening the muscles in a static manner without putting strain on the discs (see pp. 73–6). These movements are appropriate for children as well.

The lumbar curve

The posterior concavity in this region is termed lordosis and is normal. *Excessive* lordosis is pathological and is termed "hollow back" or "saddle back." Lumbar lordosis is often confused with anteversion of the pelvis. You should distinguish between the shape of the bones themselves and the external appearance of the region. An individual with large buttocks and/or prominent stomach may seem to have an accentuated lumbar curve (see *AOM*, p. 31).

There are several factors that contribute to arching of the back:
- curved alignment of the bones
- overall bodily shape and proportions
- position of the pelvis
- muscular traction
- possible psychological factors
  (which are outside the scope of this book).

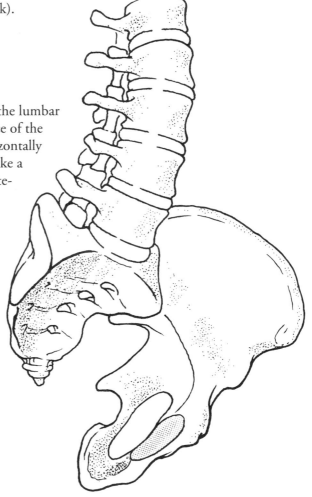

The structure of the pelvis contributes to the lumbar curve. The large, flattened, superior surface of the sacrum ("sacral base") is not oriented horizontally like a shelf, but rather is tilted anteriorly like a slide (see *AOM*, p. 47). L5, the lowest vertebra, articulates with the sacral base via a large intervertebral disc. Both L5 and the disc are thicker at the front than at the back. All of these factors contribute to the posterior concavity of the lumbar spine.

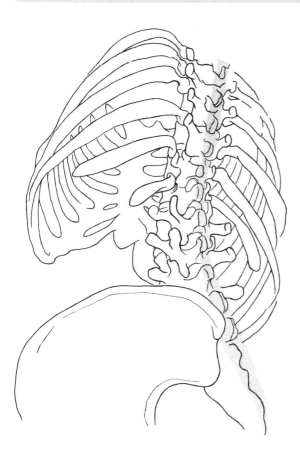

This lumbar curve continues upward and eventually gives way to the posterior convexity of the thoracic region.

The degree of curvature, and the exact level of the transition to convexity, vary depending on a person's body shape, weight distribution, center of gravity, etc. For example, in two people of the same height, the one with a longer trunk and shorter legs will have a center of gravity located at a higher vertebral level than the other person, and the lumbar curves will be correspondingly different.

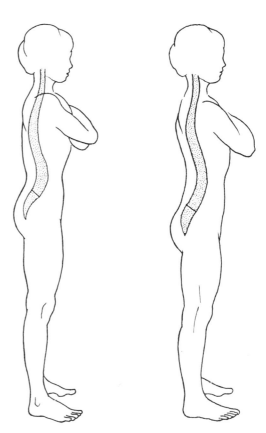

Relation of the lumbar curve to the position of the pelvis

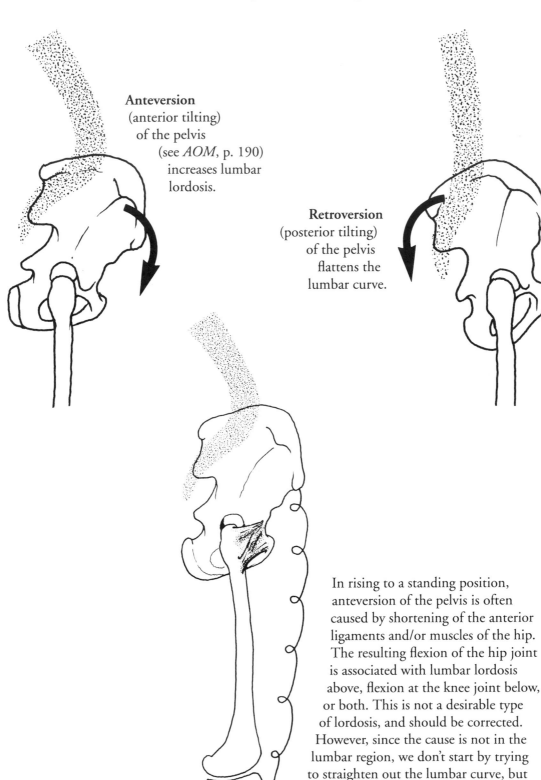

Anteversion
(anterior tilting)
of the pelvis
(see *AOM*, p. 190)
increases lumbar
lordosis.

Retroversion
(posterior tilting)
of the pelvis
flattens the
lumbar curve.

In rising to a standing position,
anteversion of the pelvis is often
caused by shortening of the anterior
ligaments and/or muscles of the hip.
The resulting flexion of the hip joint
is associated with lumbar lordosis
above, flexion at the knee joint below,
or both. This is not a desirable type
of lordosis, and should be corrected.
However, since the cause is not in the
lumbar region, we don't start by trying
to straighten out the lumbar curve, but
rather by stretching the hip in extension
(see hip flexibility exercises, pp. 158–61).

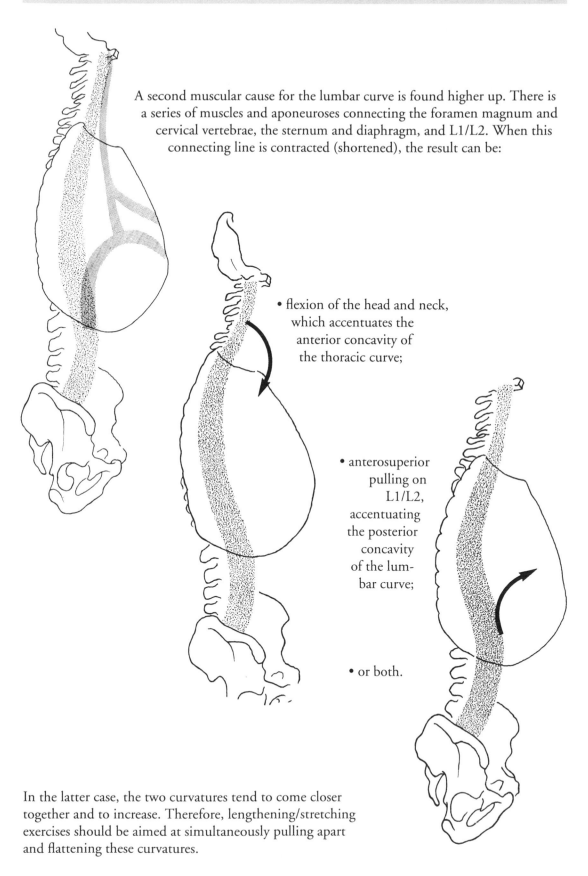

A second muscular cause for the lumbar curve is found higher up. There is a series of muscles and aponeuroses connecting the foramen magnum and cervical vertebrae, the sternum and diaphragm, and L1/L2. When this connecting line is contracted (shortened), the result can be:

• flexion of the head and neck, which accentuates the anterior concavity of the thoracic curve;

• anterosuperior pulling on L1/L2, accentuating the posterior concavity of the lumbar curve;

• or both.

In the latter case, the two curvatures tend to come closer together and to increase. Therefore, lengthening/stretching exercises should be aimed at simultaneously pulling apart and flattening these curvatures.

Flattening the lumbar curve

The lumbar curve and other curvatures of the spine are normal and beneficial. For example, they help the spine absorb shock from running and jumping, like a spring. Nonetheless, some flattening of the lumbar curve is desirable in certain physical disciplines.

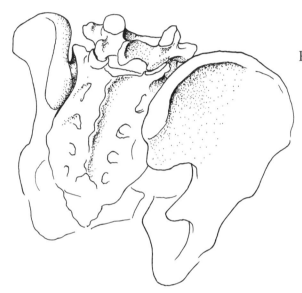

Recall that when the sacrum is sharply tilted forward, L5 tends to slide forward on the sacral base (see *AOM*, p. 51). This sliding is opposed by contact between the articular facets of S1 and the inferior articular processes of L5.

However, these processes are not designed to bear such a load; their primary job is to guide vertebral movements. If sustained, excessive loading of these processes can lead to a chain of dysfunctional events: compression, damage to the cartilage, arthrosis, local pain of ligamentary or muscular origin, edema, nerve compression, and nerve pain (in particular, sciatic pain). We thus see how sciatic pain can originate from dysfunction of bony processes, as well as from dysfunction of discs as described earlier.

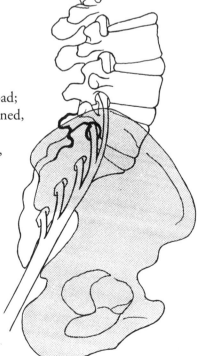

Role of the psoas and abdominal muscles

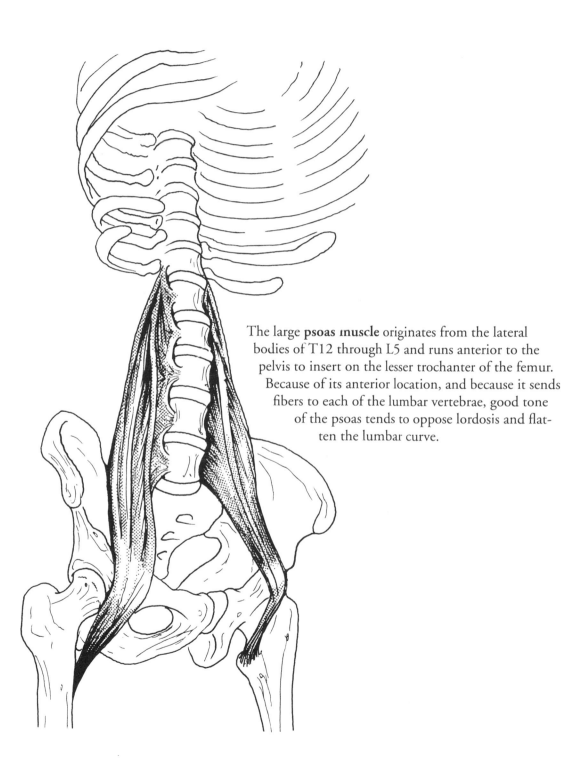

The large **psoas muscle** originates from the lateral bodies of T12 through L5 and runs anterior to the pelvis to insert on the lesser trochanter of the femur. Because of its anterior location, and because it sends fibers to each of the lumbar vertebrae, good tone of the psoas tends to oppose lordosis and flatten the lumbar curve.

Contrary to common belief, the **abdominal muscles** are not the most efficient muscles for flattening the lumbar curve. Why?

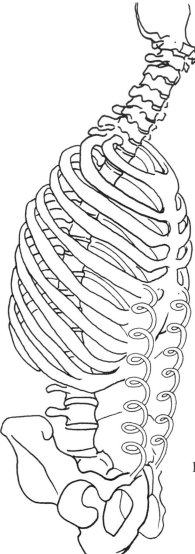

• Their attachments are to the ribs, sternum, and pelvis, not the spine. Their primary actions are to compress the abdominal contents or move the ribcage in relation to the pelvis. Their effect on the spine is therefore indirect.

• The most efficient of the abdominals, the **rectus abdominis**, pulls the sternum toward the symphysis pubis, and thereby flexes the trunk. However, in the lumbar region, the point that bends most readily is the T12-L1 hinge, which will preferentially flex before the lumbar spine does.

• Another proper role of the abdominals is to synchronize with the diaphragm in regulation of vigorous breathing.

• Sustained contraction of the abdominals in an attempt to flatten the lumbar curve may have an undesirable effect: by pulling down on the lower ribs, it tends to "collapse" the ribcage, interfere with normal breathing, and restrict ROM of the thoracic region.

Conclusion

When dealing with unwanted or excessive curvature of the lumbar spine, we need to stretch the muscular or ligamentary "brakes" which contribute to the condition. We also need to strengthen the psoas muscle to flatten the lumbar curve from the anterior side (see p. 171), or (not so effective) strengthen the abdominal muscles (see p. 68). Aside from these general guidelines, each individual lumbar curve should be evaluated in its own context. Ideally, each person should be able to arch his/her back without significant discomfort.

Thoracic region

Movements of the thoracic vertebrae cannot be dissociated from those of the ribs. In particular, the intervertebral mobilities of T1-T7 are restricted because these vertebrae are connected to "true" ribs which articulate directly to the sternum anteriorly. T8-T12 are connected to false or floating ribs and therefore have greater mobility. The ribs articulate with the sternum via costal cartilages.

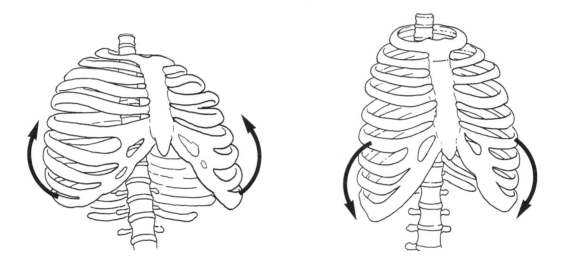

During breathing the ribs move in two different directions, each involving different articulations with the thoracic cage. The lateral movement of the ribs (called the "bucket handle" movement) causes the thorax to expand and widen.

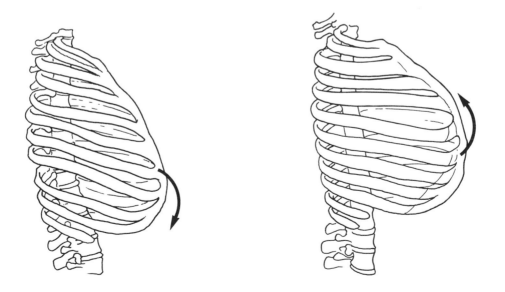

The antero-posterior movement of the sternum that accompanies inhalation and exhalation (called the "pump handle" movement) causes a narrowing of the thorax with an increase in its antero-posterior diameter.

Cervical region

Like the lumbar region, the cervical region is concave posteriorly, and the external appearance may not precisely reflect the actual alignment of the vertebrae. We like to divide the cervical region into three subregions.

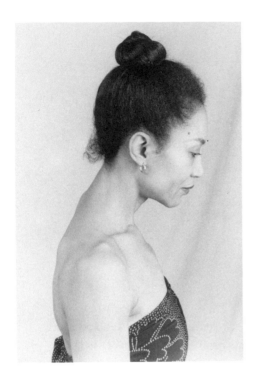

1. C7-T1 hinge

The neck is typically flexed forward here. The flexion should not be confused with the protrusion of the C7 spinous process, nor with the adipose "hump" often seen here. This flexion of the neck results mainly from:

- the series of muscles and aponeuroses described and illustrated on p. 35;

- the **sternocleidomastoid**, a large muscle originating from the sternum and clavicle and inserting on the mastoid process. When contracted bilaterally, it flexes the neck.

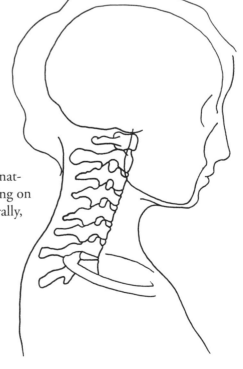

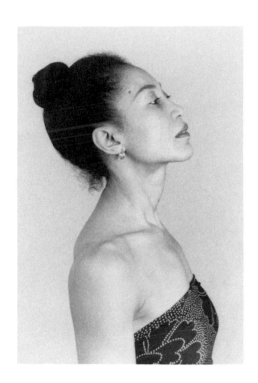

2. The neck subregion

We observe two tendencies here:

- an excessively straight holding of the head;
- more frequently, a curvature of the cervical spine which slightly reduces the height of the neck.

The spinous processes of these vertebrae vary in length. Those of C2, C6, and (particularly) C7 are long. Those of C3, C5, and (particularly) C4 are short. If we draw a line linking the tips of these processes, it is concave (and fairly irregular) posteriorly. It is along this concavity that the posterior muscles of the neck run. A line drawn connecting the anterior surfaces of the vertebrae is convex and smooth. The muscles most responsible for maintaining the cervical curvature are:

- superior trapezius
- splenius cervicis
- levator scapulae.

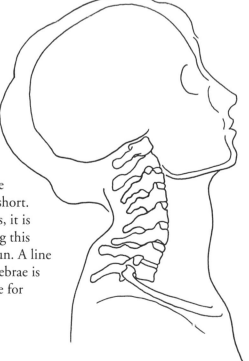

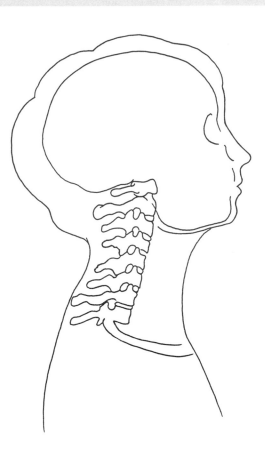

3. Skull-C1 hinge

The skull "rests" on C1 (the atlas). The front of the head is heavier than the back, but the consequent tendency of the head to drop forward is constantly opposed by tonic contraction of the posterior neck muscles.

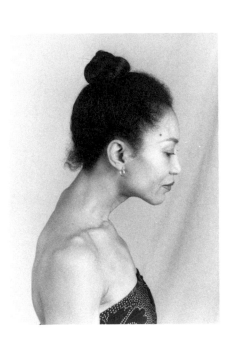

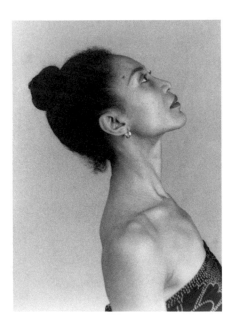

Depending on the balance of these opposing forces, we may have chronic flexion or extension of the head.

Extension of the head is accomplished by all the posterior neck muscles which insert on the skull, particularly the superior trapezius, sternocleidomastoid, and suboccipitals.

Specific exercises for three muscles are useful for supporting the cervical spine:

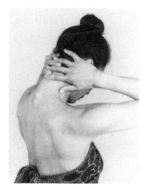

1. Semispinalis cervicis. Helps maintain the neck upright on the thorax. Crosses the back of the C7-T1 hinge and can thus elevate it. Place your hands on the posterior neck and press against the middle (C4/C5) so as to flex the neck forward.

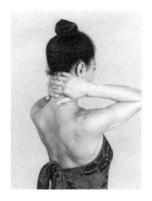

Next, move your neck back into an upright position, pushing against your hands. *Caution:* This muscle does not attach to the skull. Do not press on nor thrust the head backward during this exercise.

2. Longus colli. Can reduce cervical lordosis. As with semispinalis, first press your hands against the C4/C5 area (this time on the side of the neck instead of the back) so that the neck flexes forward, then press backward with the neck against the hands. Again, this muscle does not attach to the skull and therefore does not move the head on the neck. You need to straighten up the neck by itself without tucking in the chin.

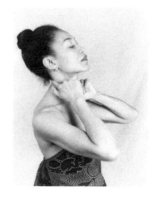

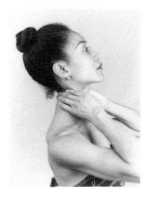

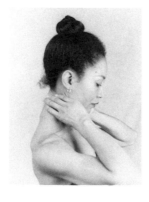

3. Suboccipital and precervical muscles. Place hands against neck as shown, such that both neck and hands are exerting pressure against each other, and move head repeatedly in nodding motion (alternate flexion/extension). This exercise helps maintain a well balanced cervical spine, characterized by strength in the lower part and good mobility in the upper part.

Practice pages: Trunk and neck

Stretching (longitudinal)*

For all stretching exercises the body should be off-load. Increase of strength is not our goal here. Rather, we are seeking to improve or maximize ROM.

Longitudinal stretching is a fundamental and very beneficial exercise, so we will give abundant explanation and direction. The purpose is to *give the intervertebral discs an opportunity to be aligned and off-load.*

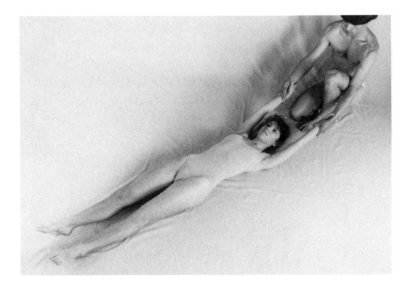

These exercises must be done on a "non-skid" mat or floor surface. Essentially, we will be pulling the sacrum and the occiput away from each other and thereby increasing the distance between successive vertebrae. As mentioned earlier, supple areas such as the T12-L1 hinge and cervical region offer less resistance to stretching than stiff areas such as the upper thoracic spine. We can utilize the non-skid property of the mat to "hold the stretch" as we move sequentially from one area to the next.

The basic exercise for **stretching of the posterior spine** is as follows:

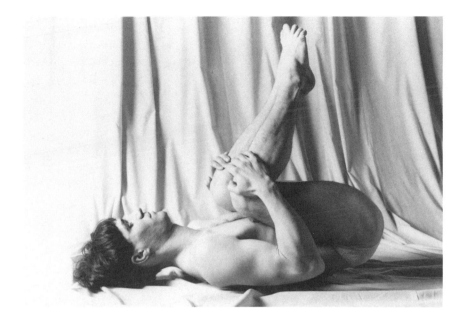

Lie on your back. Bend your knees and draw them toward the chest to stretch the lumbar vertebrae.

Place your feet back on the floor one after the other, keeping the knees bent and the entire lumbar back in contact with the floor.

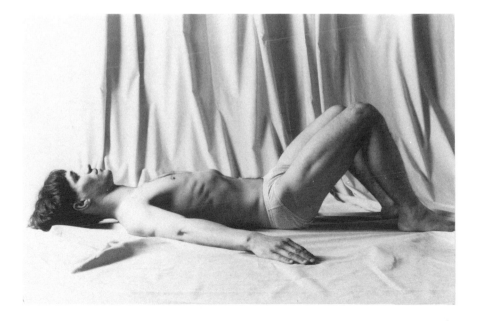

The lumbar back and pelvis must stay in constant contact with the floor throughout the remainder of this exercise.

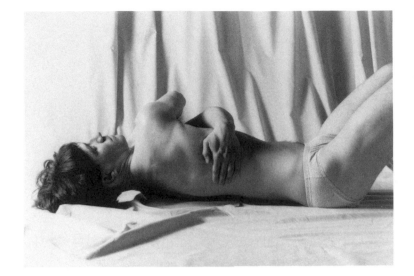

Lay your arms across the chest and clutch the ribs posteriorly. Rocking slightly from side to side, try to elongate the spine.

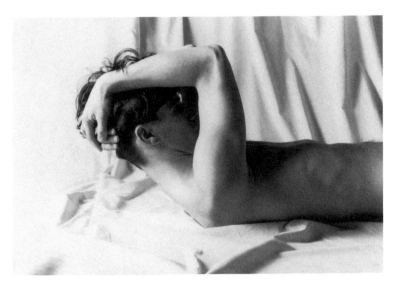

Move your hands to the back of the head and pull forward to lengthen the cervical spine.

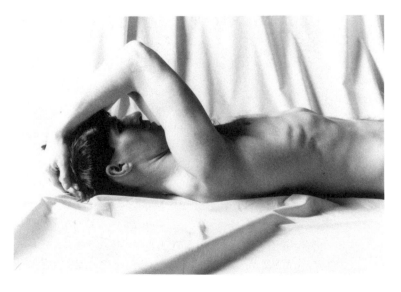

Slowly lower your head to the floor.

You can be assisted in this exercise by a partner. In particular, The thoracic region in particular is the most difficult to stretch. Your partner can help by pulling the ribs first to the right, then to the left, level after level, to gradually elongate the thoracic spine. However, to avoid straining his own lower back, your partner must keep his knees flexed, not extended.

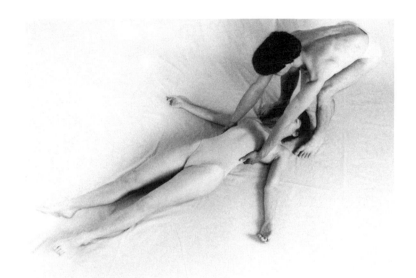

Correct position

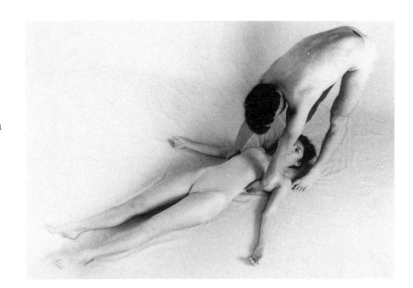

Incorrect position

Stretching of the anterior spine can be added to the preceding exercise. A good non-skid mat is essential. This exercise will have no effect if you try to do it on a slippery floor.

Starting from the last position of the preceding exercise, extend the legs by pushing the heels away,

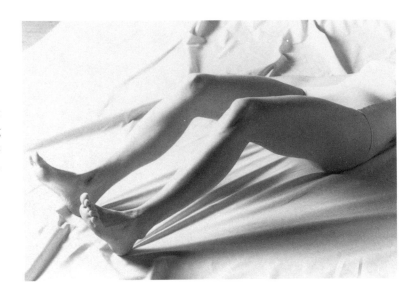

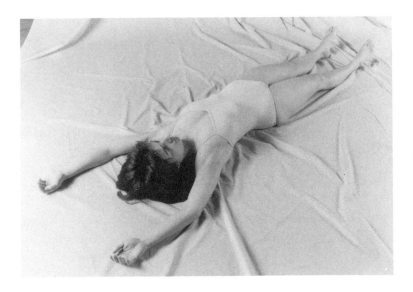

then extend the arms above the head.

Hold this position for a few minutes. During the pause, you (or your student) can work on breathing or on arm movements.

Let us look more closely at the longitudinal stretching exercise, region by region, including the legs and arms.

LUMBAR SPINE

There are several ways of simultaneously stretching the lumbar spine and placing it on the floor:

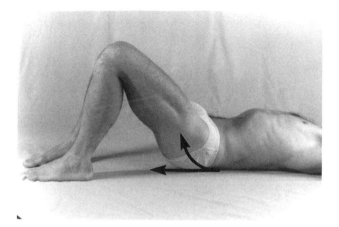

- Lie on your back such that the lumbar spine is elongated and its lordosis decreased. Accompany this movement with mini-rotations of the spine, as if crawling on one side and then the other.

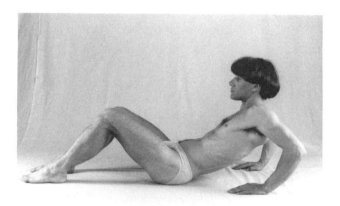

- With your weight supported by the hands and feet, lift the pelvis and lumbar spine above the floor and place them down gradually. Use a "pulling" action from the leg and arm muscles to stretch each vertebra as much as possible before placing it down.

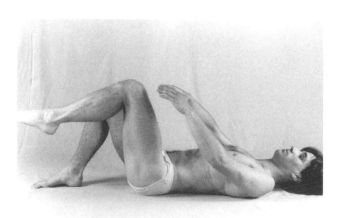

- Pull one knee, then the other, toward the chest. As you do this, concentrate on stretching the lumbar vertebrae apart from each other.

THORACIC SPINE

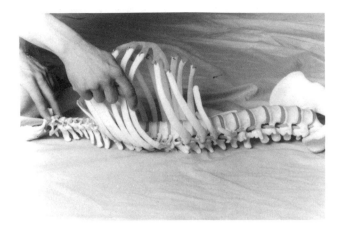

Enlarging the intercostal spaces helps stretch the vertebrae.

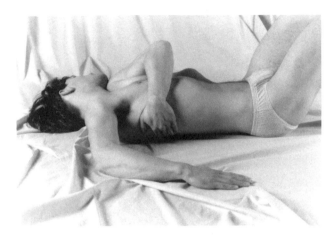

For example, turn slightly to the left, grab the right ribs with your hand, lift the T12-T11 intercostal space to open it up, breathe into this space, then lower it onto the non-skid floor, where it should stay "open." Try to prevent it from returning to its original position when you do the same exercise on the opposite side. In this manner, work alternately on the left and right sides, space by space, along the entire thoracic spine.

You can also have a partner do the lifting and stretching of the ribs. To protect her back, the partner should keep knees bent and one hand on the floor for support.

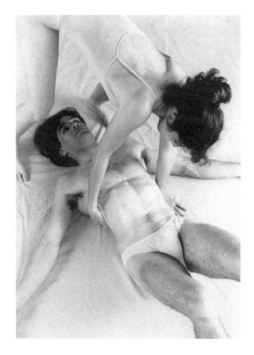

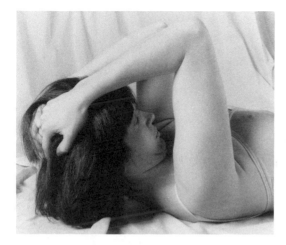

CERVICAL SPINE

We wish to avoid excessive flexing at the C1-occiput . . .

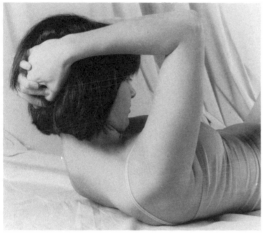

. . . or T1-C7 joints, which are already hypermobile hinge areas.

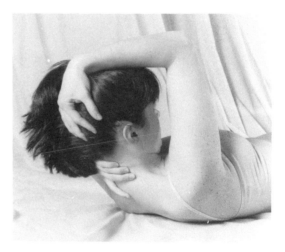

Instead, stretch the neck from the back by massaging with your (or your partner's) hand along the muscle masses that you can feel on either side of the spinous processes. Do this alternately on the right and left, placing the neck down as you go.

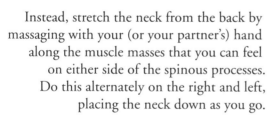

When the head is finally about to touch the floor, pull gently at the hair so as to place the head as far as possible from the shoulders and maintain the stretch of the cervical spine.

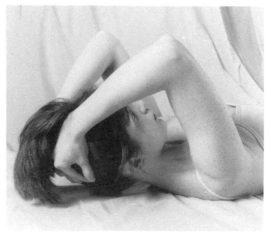

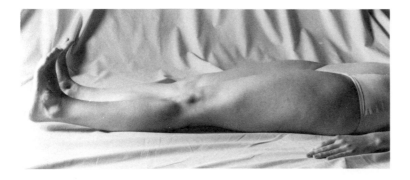

LEGS

Lengthen them one at a time. Push each heel (slightly raised off the floor) as far away as possible,

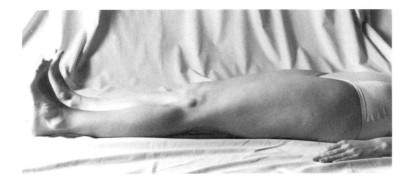

then lower it to the floor.

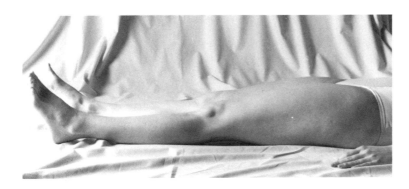

Release (plantar flex) the anterior part of the foot.

This exercise takes the pelvis into anteversion, and the lumbar spine into lordosis, stretching the lumbar vertebrae apart anteriorly.

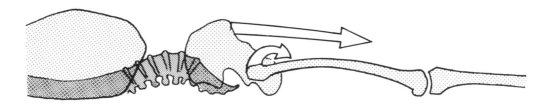

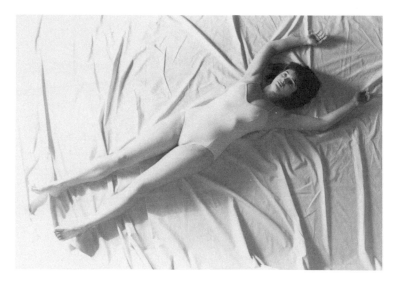

ARMS

Stretch the arms above the head, concentrating on one at a time. Your partner can help you by pulling gently.

This exercise activates the latissimus dorsi and pectoralis major, causing an opening of the costal spaces and lordosis at the thoracic/lumbar spinal level. This lordosis is combined with the lower lumbar lordosis. However, this combined "arch" does not have a shortening effect if the head-sacrum distance has remained long (because of the non-slip flooring) during the exercise.

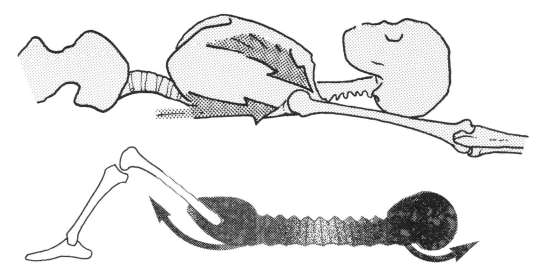

We can think of the entire spine as an "accordion" which has been stretched first from the back,

and then from the front.

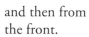

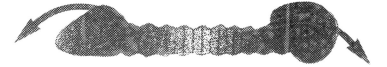

If this exercise is done for prolonged periods, you should support the lordosis by placing a small cushion or rolled up towel under the lumbar vertebrae.

Two additional longitudinal stretching exercises:

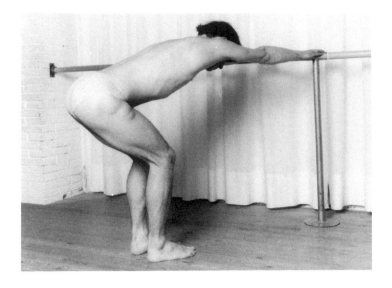

- Place both hands on a bar, and step back so that the pelvis is as far away as possible from the wall and the back is like a long, flat table. Your partner can help by pulling the pelvis back.

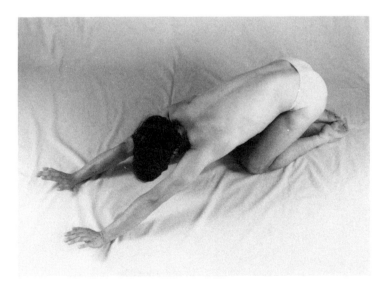

- Kneel with the hands on the floor as far forward as possible, and stretch the buttocks back as if trying to rest them on the heels. The head is aligned with the back.

In both these exercises, the spine is stretched in its entirety with no distinction between different areas or types of mobility. They are simpler but less precise than the preceding exercises. Don't try them if you have pain or restrictions in the shoulders.

Stretching with bending

These exercises stretch the spine not with a head to sacrum elongation, but with a curving action which makes one side (the one to be stretched) more convex, and the other more concave.

FORWARD BENDS

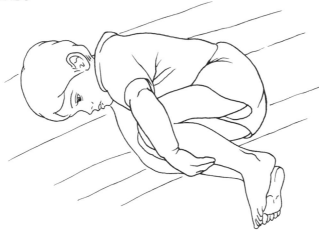

Lie down on the floor on one side.

Forward-bend the spine by holding either the head or the knees with your hands.

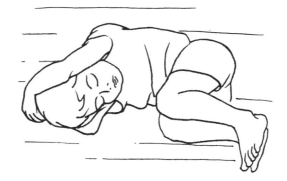

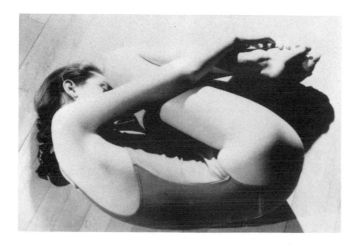

You can use breathing techniques to make the convex side bigger. Inhale "in the back" of the ribs, and use exhalation to close the front even more.

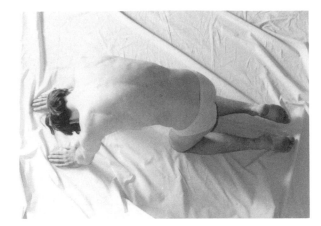

You can also do forward-bending while supporting your weight on the hands and knees. This produces a slightly heavier load on the vertebrae.

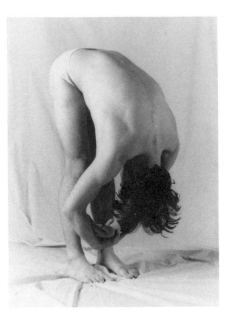

Some people forward-bend from a standing position, with no support from the hands. We do not recommend this. It does stretch the back muscles, but at the cost of heavy compression of the lumbar vertebral disks.

BACKBENDS

Lie on one side and extend the spine backward. Adult students can support the head with a small cushion or the arm. Inhale "in the front" of the ribs to open them, or allow the abdomen to expand during inhalation. Since the spine is off-load in this exercise, it is generally not harmful to try for extreme ROM (backward curvature). However, individuals with lower back problems or sciatic nerve dysfunction should be cautious, or avoid this exercise.

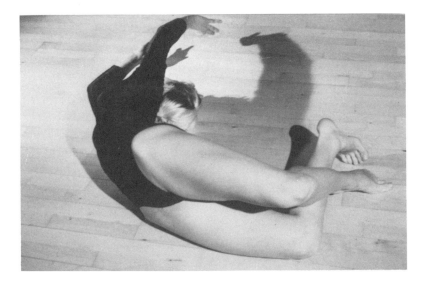

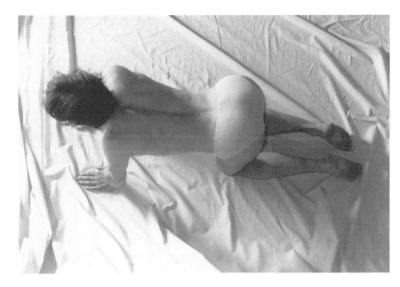

You can also arch the back from a hands and knees position.

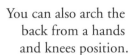

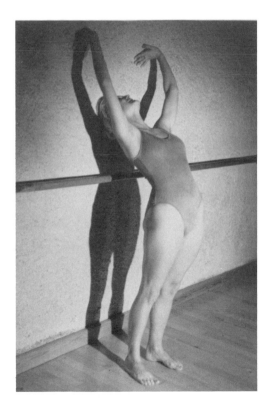

Another alternative is to stand close to a wall, back to it, legs slightly apart. Lift your arms above the head, press the hands against the wall, and lift the sternum up and forward.

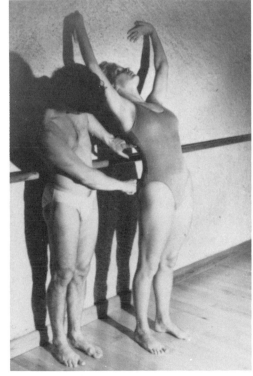

Concentrate on arching the spine at the thoracic region, not just at the more flexible lumbar region. A partner can help with this.

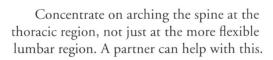

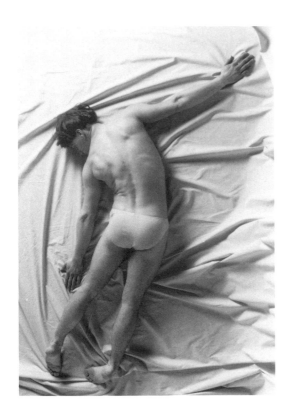

SIDEBENDS

Lie either on the back or front. Bend sideways so that the left shoulder or ear moves closer to the left thigh. If lying on your back, keep the pelvis and shoulder blades in contact with the floor. If you have no shoulder problems, add a right arm movement above the head which will promote opening of the right ribs.

You can even pull the right hand with the left one. Repeat this process for the opposite side. To further increase the opening on the convex side, try crossing one foot over the other.

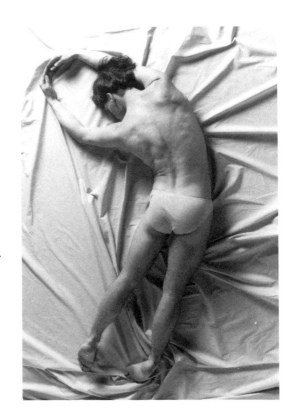

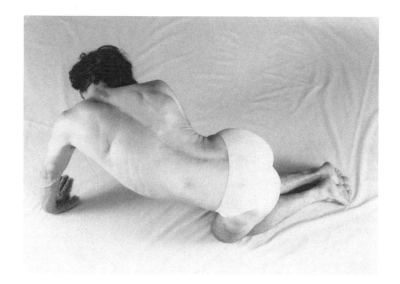

Sidebending can also be done on the hands and knees,

with the option of adding on extension or flexion,

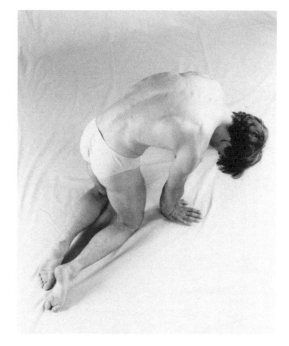

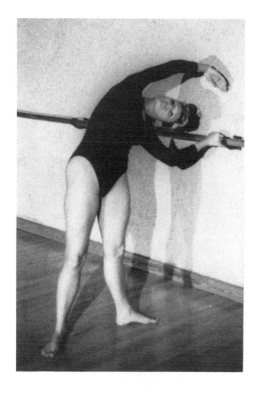

or in a standing position, with one hand firmly holding the bar for support. In these positions, always be aware of where the movement is occurring. As we have seen, some parts of the spine are much more flexible than others. An off-load situation is the best time to observe the hypermobile areas without danger, and to learn how to intentionally limit movement at specific areas, through contraction of opposing muscles. This is excellent preparation for coordination exercises (see p. 77).

Stretching with spinal rotations

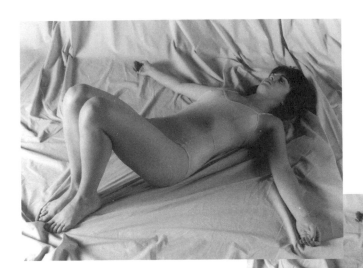

Lie on your back,
arms stretched
outward, knees bent.

Keeping the legs in
contact, twist the
pelvis so that the
knees touch (or
almost touch) the
floor on one side.

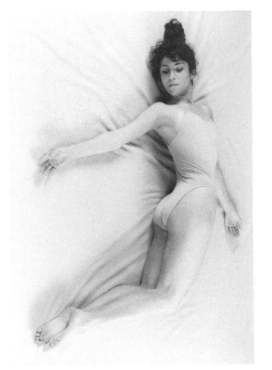

You can alter the level where twisting occurs
(move it superiorly) by keeping the shoulders
in contact with the floor, further twisting
the lower body as shown, and pushing the
knees farther away from the head.

Roll back to a supine position, maintaining
the stretch, then perform the same movement
on the opposite side.

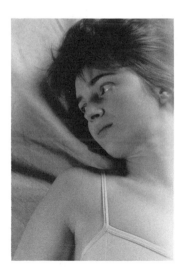

Twist your head to one side and then the other. Always return to the center.

Finally, combine these two exercises, twisting the knees to the right and the head to the left, then vice versa.

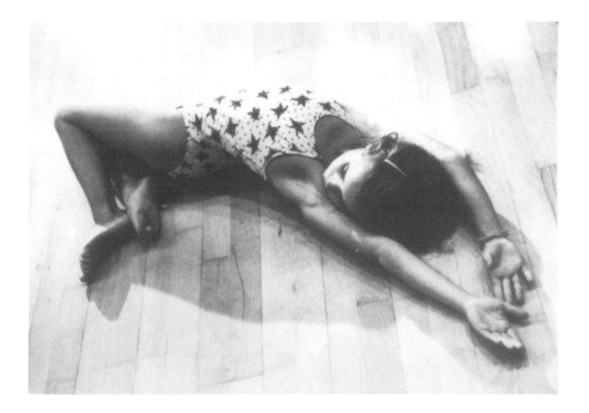

The advice given above for bending exercises also applies to these twisting (rotation) movements. These off-load exercises provide a good opportunity to locate the hypermobile areas of the spine, and to learn to prevent excessive movement there through localized action of the opposing rotator muscles.

Strengthening deep muscles

We are typically unaware of the deep spinal muscles. A partner can help us "awaken" them.

TACTILE STIMULATION*

Your partner pokes suddenly and strongly into the muscle mass on either side of the spine. Allow yourself to react spontaneously to this.

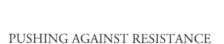

PUSHING AGAINST RESISTANCE

Your partner presses downward against your head. You resist this through contraction of the neck and spinal muscles.

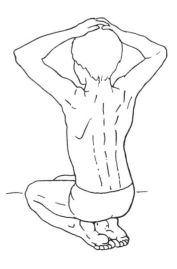

You can perform a similar exercise without a partner: push down with both hands against the head, and simultaneously use the neck muscles to push upward against this resistance, as if trying to lengthen the neck.

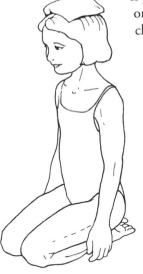

If you enjoy balancing objects on your head, you can even use a beanbag or small bag of rice to provide the resistance and awaken the deep muscles. Make sure the object is not so heavy as to cause any discomfort.

By pushing the knees (alternately) against the hands, you can strengthen the psoas muscles. At the same time, try to flatten the lumbar curvature against the floor.

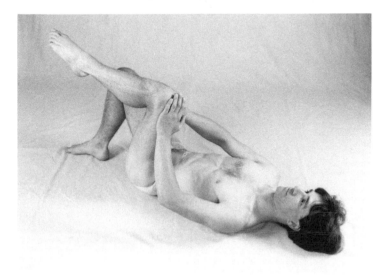

To strengthen longissimus cervicis, a long muscle of the neck, elongate and straighten the neck.

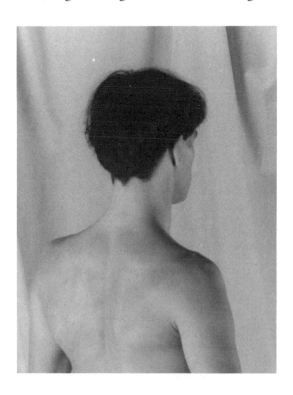

Don't confuse this movement with "tucking in the chin" (i.e., flexing the head against some resistance).

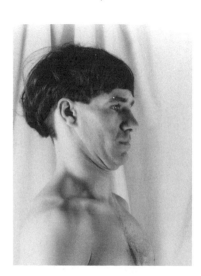

UNDULATING MOVEMENTS

Lie down on the floor on one side, hips and knees flexed. Try arching (extending) the spine one intervertebral space at a time. Start with the lower lumbar region where this is easiest to do, then gradually work upward, trying to produce a similar movement at each level.

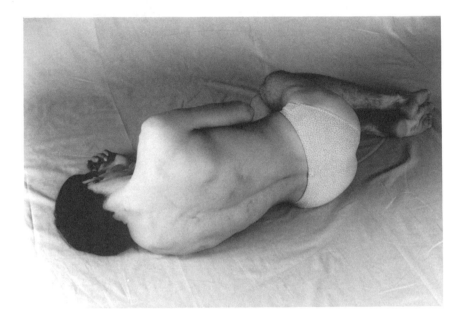

Next, try to *flex* the spine one intervertebral space at a time. Start at the lower thoracic region where this is easiest, then work gradually through the other areas.

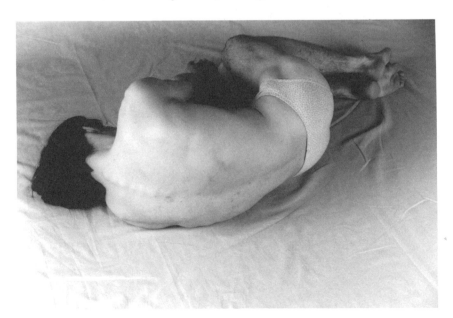

After you become familiar with these movements, you can try combining them into a continuous undulatory movement, like a wave traveling along a string. The shoulders and pelvis will follow this action, but not initiate it.

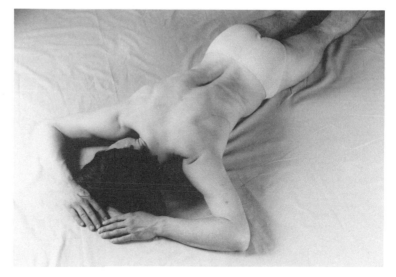

You can do this in a prone or elbow/knee position,

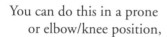
seated position,

supine position,

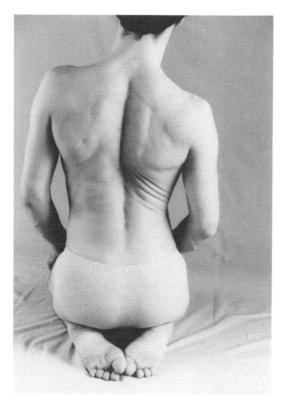

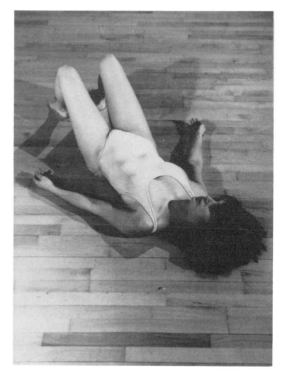

or standing with hips and knees bent. This undulatory movement can be further combined with small lateral movements or rotations of the spine. After this type of exercise, you may feel sensations of heat along the spine, which shows that the deep muscles are working.

Strengthening superficial muscles

POSTERIOR MUSCLES.

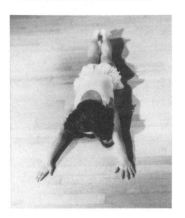

Lie face down on the floor, legs straight and close together. Stretch out the arms and neck, with palms and forehead slightly raised off the floor.

Turn the palms upward.

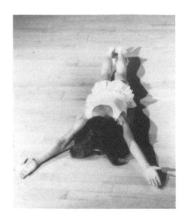

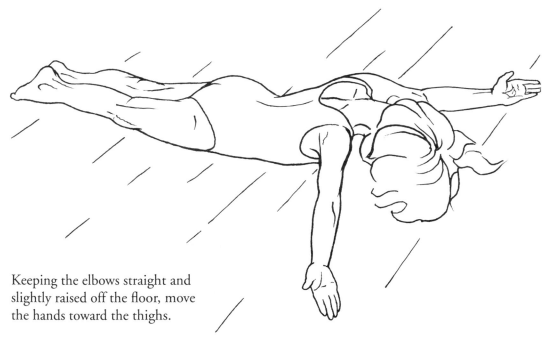

Keeping the elbows straight and slightly raised off the floor, move the hands toward the thighs.

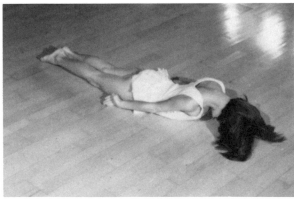

When the hands touch the thighs, drop them to the floor, rest a moment, then return to the starting position.

More muscles can be brought into play by elevating the head and/or legs during this exercise.

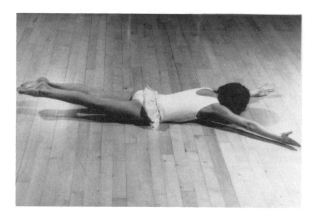

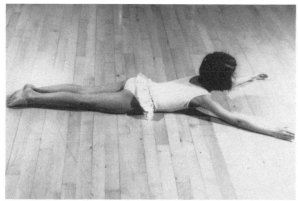

Lifting the head works the superior **trapezius**.

Lifting the arms off the floor involves the **latissimus dorsi** in addition to the trapezius.

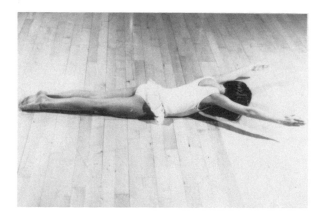

Lifting the legs works the **gluteus** muscles in addition to the latissimus dorsi and large gluteal muscles.

During this exercise, you will feel sensations of heat from the entire back, since you are using the large superficial muscles as well as deep muscles.

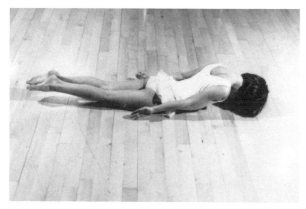

ABDOMINAL MUSCLES

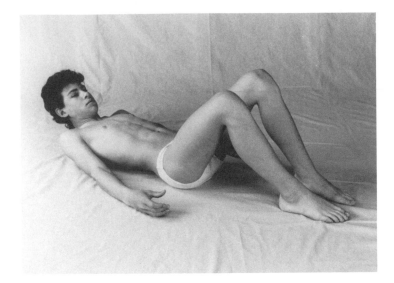

Lie on your back with knees bent, and lift the head. This activates the **rectus abdominis** muscles. By inhaling deeply at the same time, you also activate the **transversus abdominis**.

Twisting the shoulders alternately to either side activates the abdominal **obliques**.

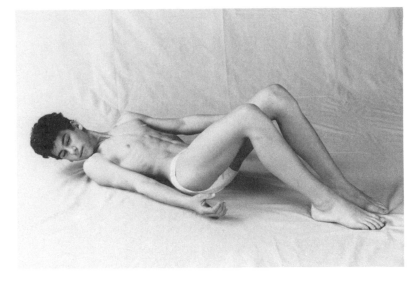

In these exercises, the abdominal muscles bring the ribs closer to the pelvis. The flexors of the neck attach to the ribs or sternum. To hold the ribs, we "fasten" them to the pubis through contraction (isometric) of the rectus abdominis, which simultaneously calls into play the neck flexors (isotonic contraction). This is an example of a "muscular chain."

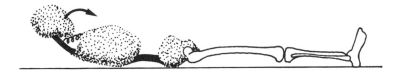

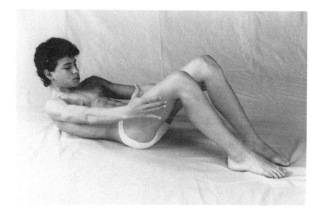

Next, flex the trunk so as to bring the shoulder girdle and rib cage toward the knees. Now the contraction of the neck flexors is isometric, and that of the rectus abdominis is isotonic.

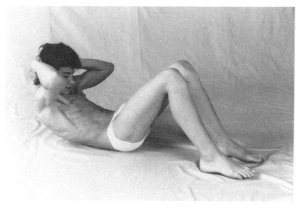

This exercise can be made even more demanding by placing the hands behind the head, which effectively increases the weight being lifted.

Similarly, the exercise becomes easier as the head is held farther forward,

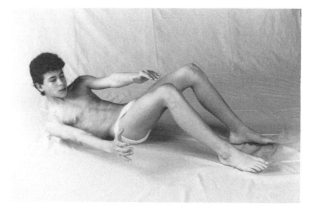

and more difficult as the head is held farther back.

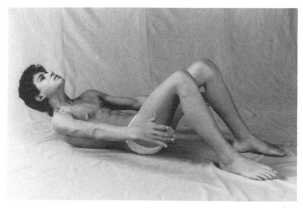

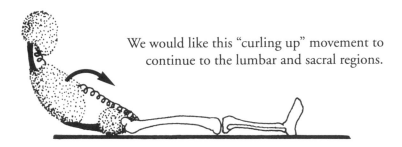

We would like this "curling up" movement to continue to the lumbar and sacral regions.

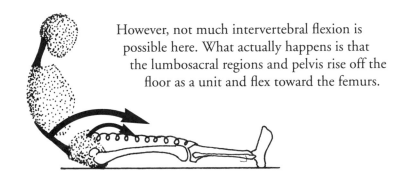

However, not much intervertebral flexion is possible here. What actually happens is that the lumbosacral regions and pelvis rise off the floor as a unit and flex toward the femurs.

The muscles responsible for this are not the abdominals but the **hip flexors** (psoas, iliacus, and rectus femoris). If the pelvis were fixed, these muscles would flex the femurs. In the present case, however, the femurs are fixed and the pelvis is being moved.

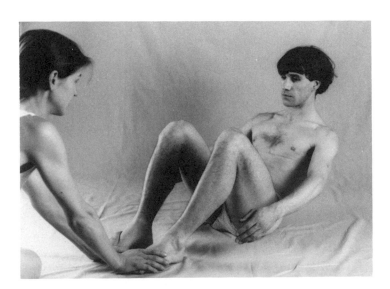

Some people will need their feet held in place to complete this exercise;

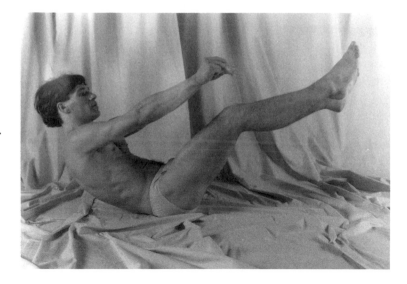

otherwise, their feet come off the floor and they fall backward.

The problem here is not lack of spinal mobility nor abdominal muscle strength, but rather insufficient counterbalance resulting from physical proportions: the weight of the lower limbs is not sufficient to counteract the weight of the trunk. People with a short trunk and long legs can easily do this exercise without assistance.

People with a long trunk and short legs who try to do this exercise without help will generally resort to one of two strategies:
• Use kinetic energy to "throw" the arms, head, and trunk forward.
• Use trunk muscles rather than hip flexors to bring the trunk forward. This "forces" spinal flexion at the most mobile points: the thoracic/lumbar and lumbar/sacral junctions. Stressing these junctions is a bad idea. Instead, find a partner to hold down your feet, or hook the feet under the bottom of a couch.

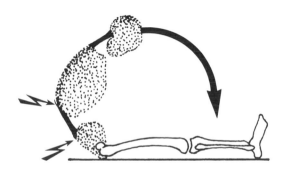

As an alternative to keeping the feet on the ground and lifting the trunk, you can keep the trunk on the ground and lift the feet. This is the most commonly used exercise for strengthening the abdominal muscles. Obviously, the muscles responsible for lifting the legs here are not the abdominals but the hip flexors. However, the abdominals are contracted in order to fix and stabilize the pelvis. The hip flexors tend to antevert the pelvis and arch the lower back; the abdominals counteract this.

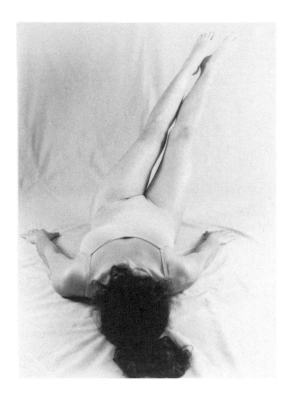

You can maximally activate the abdominals by raising both legs simultaneously and keeping the knees straight.

Progressive degrees of difficulty are shown here:
- easiest: one leg at a time lifted, knee flexed;
- intermediate: both legs lifted, held straight up, knees straight;
- hardest: both legs lifted, and held slightly off the floor.

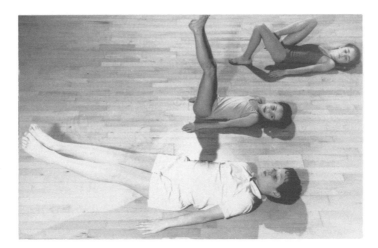

Once again, during these leg lifting exercises, you can solicit the transverse muscles by inhaling deeply, or solicit the transverse muscles by twisting the upper body to one side and the other.

People with problems of the lumbar spine should avoid the exercises on pp. 70–3, and stick with those shown on pp. 68–9.

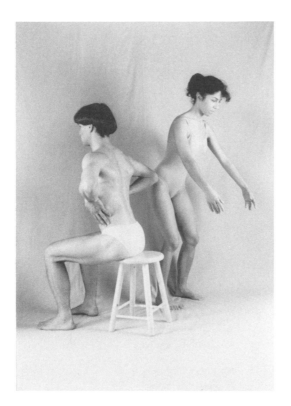

Coordination with straight spine*

Our purpose here is not to increase ROM, but to improve alignment and balance of the trunk, as a basis for more complex movements later.

For purposes of these exercises, imagine that the spine is straight and rigid from the sacrum to the occiput—and keep it that way. Sit down on the edge of a seat with your weight on the ischial tuberosities. Place your hands on the space between the ribs and pelvis, such that they touch the lower ribs and anterior superior iliac spine at the same time. These bony landmarks should stay in the same relation to each other throughout these exercises.

Tilt the straight spine forward. The posterior muscles contract (you can confirm this by placing your hands on either side of the spine). It is important to maintain:

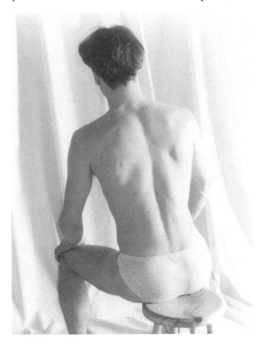

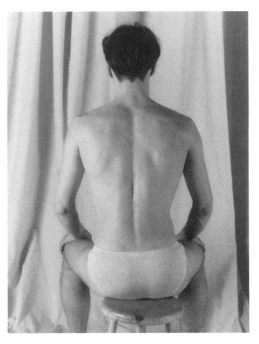

• equal pressure on the two ischia

• equal contraction of the right and left sets of posterior muscles.

Two incorrect positions are shown here:

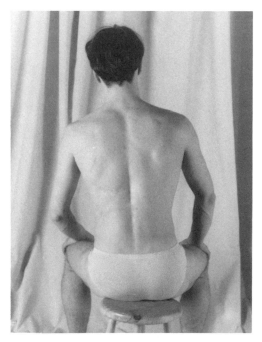

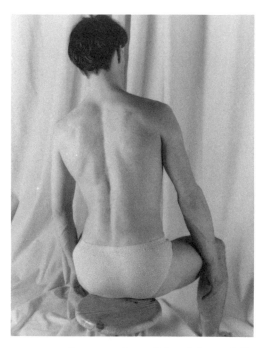

• unequal pressure on the ischia

• unequal contraction of the right vs. left posterior muscles.

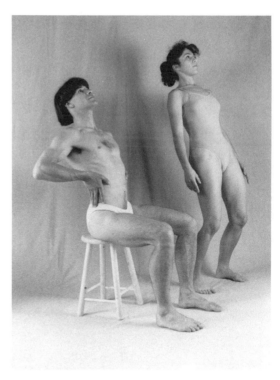

Lean the straight spine
backward. Now the
abdominal muscles
are activated.

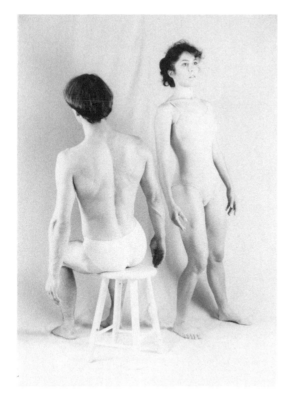

Alternately flex the right
and left knees. The straight
spine will respectively lean
to the right or left.

Combine the above exercises: forward-backward and left-right movements. Keep checking the
relative position of the bony landmarks with your hands to make sure they stay constant.

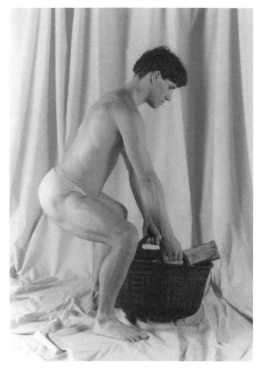

The straight spine position is the only one that is risk-free for lifting, pulling, or carrying heavy objects. With a straight spine, there is no pinching or squeezing of any intervertebral disc.

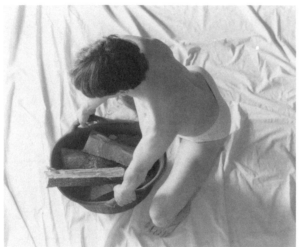

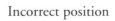

Incorrect position

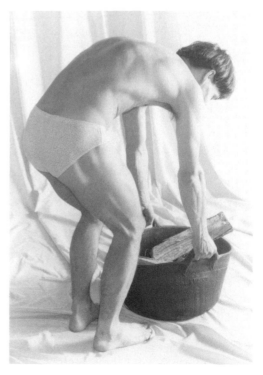

Coordination with bending

In these exercises, the spine
is bent anteriorly (flexion),

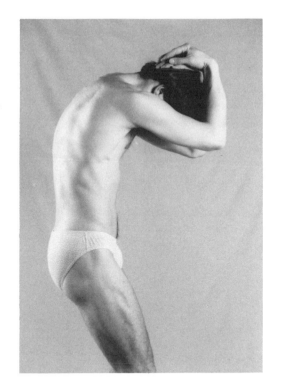

posteriorly (extension),

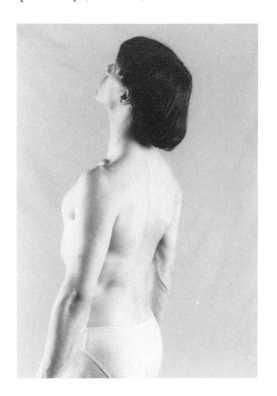

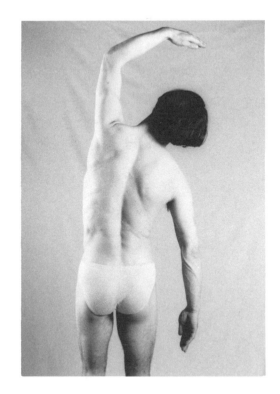

or laterally.

We are not looking for large ROM in these bending exercises. We wish to avoid compressing the discs, i.e., avoid pinching on the concave side. For this purpose, we will use the braking action of the opposing muscles on the convex side.

General principles:

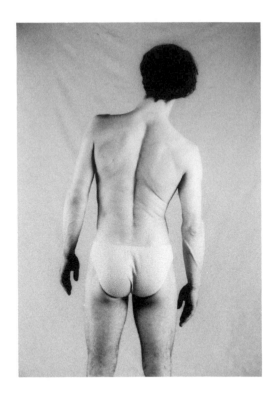

- Movements close to the
  vertical line use mostly
  the deep muscles.

- As movements get farther away from the vertical line, the superficial muscles are
  increasingly solicited.

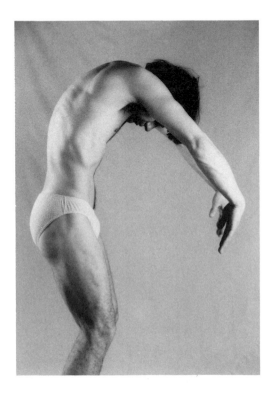

- When the arms are held
  away from the body, both
  deep and superficial muscles
  are active.

Exercises to avoid

Do *not* try to stretch the hamstrings or lumbar spine by any of the following:

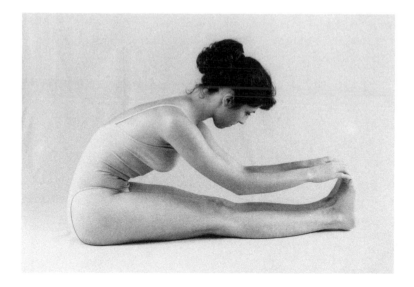

• leaning forward with straight legs

• same position, with outstretched arms

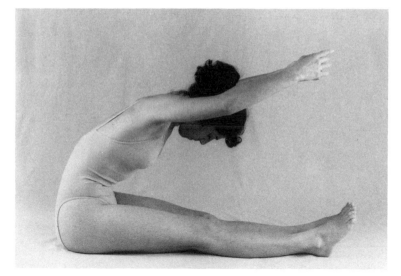

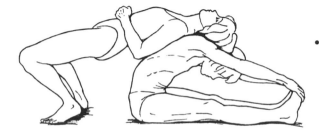

• same position, with another person leaning on your back.

All these techniques put excessive stress on the lumbar intervertebral discs. For safer stretching of the lumbar spine, see pp. 49, 55–9. For safer stretching of the hamstrings, see pp. 164–67.

Also to be avoided, for the same reason:

• Standing with straight knees and dropping the upper body forward, arms hanging down or wrapped around the knees. This is similar to the position shown on the top of p. 79. It is sometimes recommended as a way to "release" tension in (or "relax") the back. In fact, however, this position results in contraction of the posterior spinal muscles, as you can confirm by placing your hands on either side of the spine.

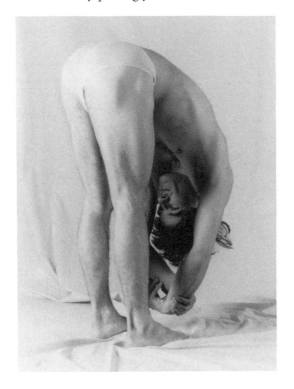
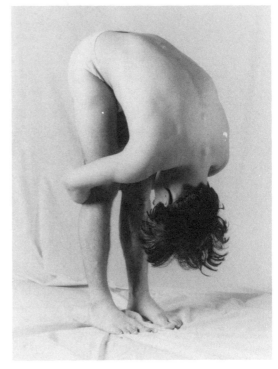

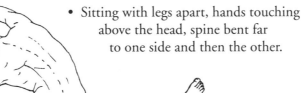

• Sitting with legs apart, hands touching above the head, spine bent far to one side and then the other.

• Sitting with legs apart, hands touching in front, spine rotated far to one side and then the other.

Again, each of these exercises puts excessive stress on the lumbar discs. There are safer ways to achieve the same results.

CHAPTER THREE

The Shoulder

....

The shoulder girdle supports the two arms, and also provides attachments for several muscles involved in movements of the head. Good mobility and coordination of the joints and muscles of the shoulder, elbow, wrist, and hand are essential for many of our day-to-day activities. Strength is important too, but less so than for the legs. In this chapter, our major emphasis will be on movement coordination.

Movements

Movements at the shoulder involve three joints:
- **sternoclavicular joint**, between sternum and clavicle
- **acromioclavicular joint**, between scapula and clavicle
- **glenohumeral joint**, between scapula and humerus.

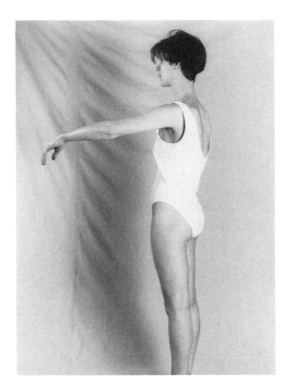

In **flexion** the arm is raised in front of the body, in a sagittal plane. This movement can reach 180°, with the arm held straight overhead. Small-scale flexion is the most common shoulder movement, as in driving a car, working at a keyboard, pressing a button, leaning on the forearms.

Extreme shoulder flexion is associated with extension of the spine.

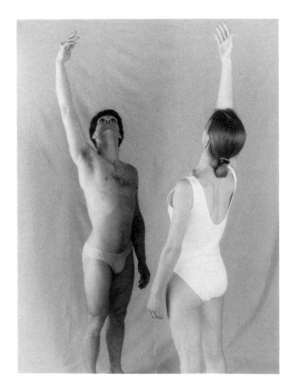

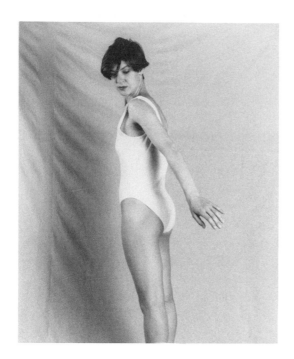

In **extension** the arm moves posterior to the body in a sagittal plane. This movement is much less common than flexion, and has a smaller ROM. Examples are leaning back on the elbows, or slamming a door behind you. Extreme shoulder extension is associated with flexion of the trunk.

In **abduction** the arm moves laterally away from the body in a frontal plane. ROM is almost 180°. This movement is more common in specific physical disciplines or exercises than in most people's everyday lives.

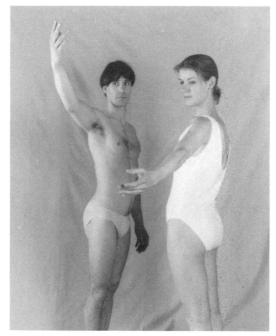

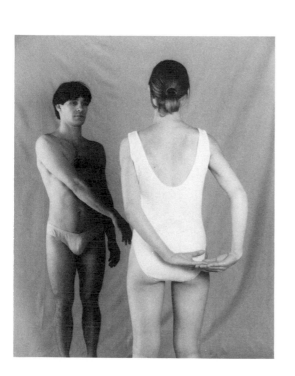

In **adduction** the arm moves medially from an abducted position back toward the body. If adduction is combined with flexion or extension, the arm can cross in front of or behind the body.

In **rotation** at the shoulder joint, the humerus turns on its own longitudinal axis. These movements can be performed with the elbow straight, but should be demonstrated and explained to students with the elbow bent; otherwise, they are easily confused with pronation and supination, a crossing of the bones of the forearm which has nothing to do with the shoulder joint.

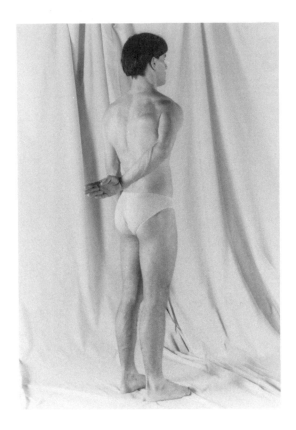

Medial rotation takes the arm into a spiral-like movement from the shoulder. In ordinary movements, ROM is about 30°. Medial rotation is often combined with flexion in movements such as catching a ball or hugging a person.

In **lateral (external) rotation** the arm is turned toward the outside, away from the body. This is a less common movement in everyday life.

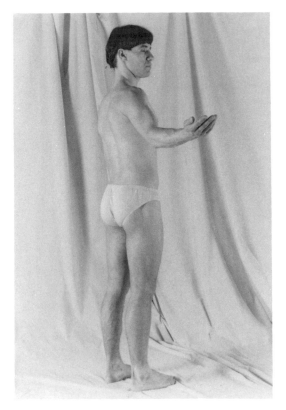

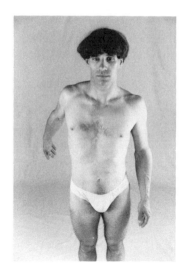

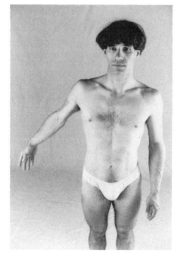

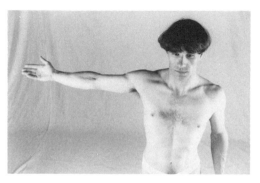

Overall, the shoulder has the greatest ROM of any joint in the body, but ROM is larger and the associated muscles stronger for movements that bring the arms forward or toward the body (flexion, adduction, medial rotation) than for the opposite movements. This becomes obvious as you move your shoulder in circumduction (a combined movement where the hand describes a very large circle in the air, and the arm describes the surface of a large cone).

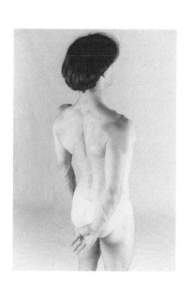

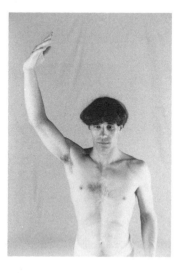

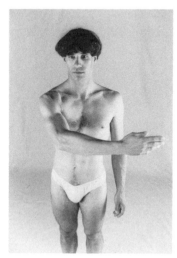

The base of this "cone" is directed much more anteriorly than posteriorly.

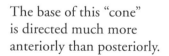

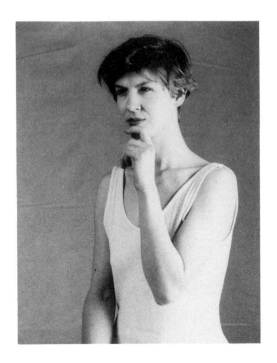

In real life the shoulder performs complex, combined movements rather than pure flexion, pure abduction, etc. For example, as you pick up food from a table at your side and bring it toward your mouth, the shoulder is undergoing combined flexion, adduction, and medial rotation.

In the standard "anatomical position" which we use as a reference in anatomy, the arms hang straight down at the sides, and the palms face anteriorly (see *AOM*, p. 1). As far as the shoulder joint is concerned, this position differs from "zero functional position" in which:
- articular facets have maximal contact
- the various ligaments and muscles of the shoulder are in a state of average and equal tension
- there is good ROM for all movements, in all directions.

In zero functional position, the shoulder shows slight flexion, slight adduction, and slight medial rotation (its three preferred movements).

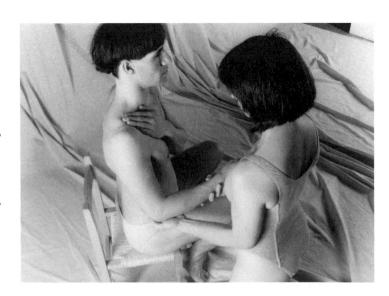

Movements of the shoulder girdle itself

So far, we have been talking mainly about movements of the humerus, i.e., movements at the glenohumeral joint. We should also mention movements of the shoulder girdle itself, which consists of the clavicle and scapula. These movements involve the sternoclavicular and acromioclavicular joints. The scapula ("shoulder blade") has many more muscle attachments than the clavicle ("collar bone"), so movements of the clavicle are generally secondary to those of the scapula.

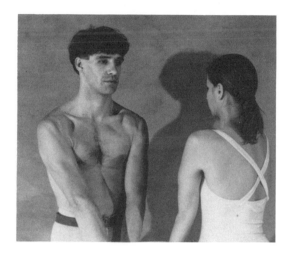

Flexion (forward movement) of the shoulder girdle is often a movement of protection or guarding. Chronic flexion is typically due to sustained contraction of the pectoralis minor or pectoralis major muscles.

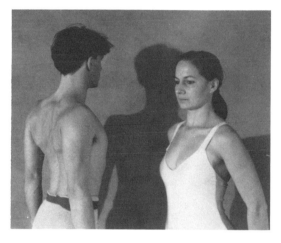

Extension (backward movement) of the shoulder girdle is commonly seen in people consciously trying to maintain an erect posture.

Elevation (upward movement) is another movement of protection, e.g., when you anticipate a blow on the head. Chronic elevation may be caused by contraction of the trapezius muscle and have psychological origins.

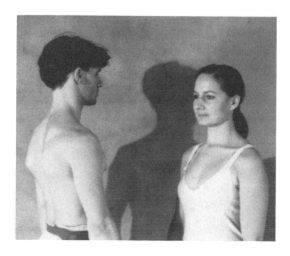

Depression (downward movement) is normally a return from elevation. It's difficult to depress the shoulder girdle much below resting position.

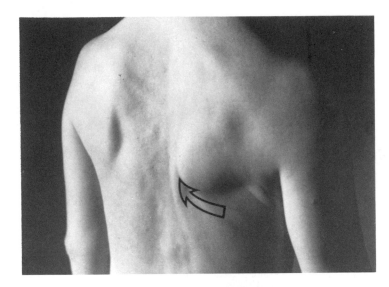

We can also speak of some movements of the scapula by itself, as it "floats" over the posterior ribcage (see also *AOM*, pp. 109–10).

In **downward rotation** the glenoid cavity moves downward, and the inferior angle of the scapula moves superomedially (see arrow in photograph).

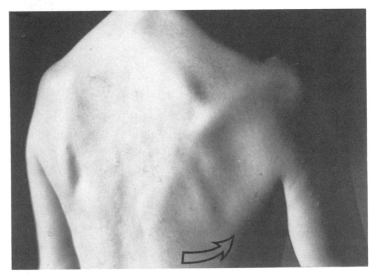

In **upward rotation** the glenoid cavity moves upward, and the inferior angle moves superolaterally (see arrow).

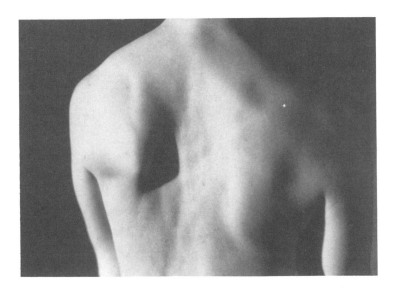

In **retraction (adduction)** the medial border of the scapula is pulled close to the spinal column by contraction of the serratus anterior muscle, and becomes indistinct (see right scapula in this photo).

In **protraction (abduction)** the medial border is pulled away from the ribcage by the infraspinatus, teres minor, and teres major muscles, and becomes more prominent (left scapula in photo).

Flexibility of the shoulder

In contrast to hinge joints such as the elbow, the glenohumeral joint of the shoulder doesn't have much in the way of bony structures acting as brakes to limit movement. Pure adduction is stopped by contact between the humerus and ribcage, and extreme abduction or flexion may be limited by contact of the humerus with the scapula, but that's all.

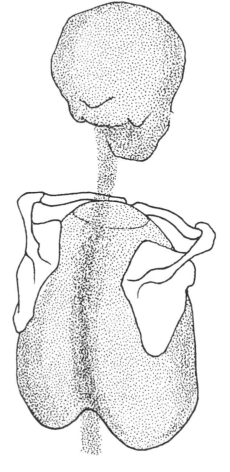

The large ROM of the glenohumeral joint is amplified by the flexibility of the shoulder girdle itself. Remember that the scapula is not attached directly to the thorax by any bony joint, but only by muscles.

Connective tissue structures such as joint capsules, ligaments, and tendons do not limit the shoulder joint nearly as much as they do the hip joint. The capsule of the glenohumeral joint is loose, offers little resistance, and has some weak points anteriorly. It is reinforced superiorly by two thickened portions (ligaments) which look like "suspenders" of the arms. They are actually not powerful enough to perform this function, but they do limit extreme flexion and extension. If flexion is combined with lateral rotation at the start, tension of the ligaments will promote medial rotation as flexion proceeds.

The loose arrangement of capsule and ligaments at the shoulder joint can be subject to inflammations (**capsulitis, periarthritis**). A condition called retractile capsulitis greatly limits some or all arm movements. This type of retractile pathology is very rare in children or teenagers.

Since limitation of shoulder movement by bony or connective tissue structures is minimal, integrity of the joint depends mainly on the surrounding muscles. Shoulder joint restrictions are often due to stiffening of shoulder muscles, or related neck muscles. Some muscles prone to stiffness are described below.

Deep muscles

The "**rotator cuff**" consists of the subscapularis, infraspinatus, supraspinatus, and teres minor muscles. They originate from various points on the scapula and all insert on the superior humerus. Their bodies surround the joint capsule, except anteroinferiorly (see *AOM*, pp. 120–22). These muscles remain partially contracted most of the time in order to support the arm, even when it is hanging "at rest" at the side of the body. The only time they can truly relax is when the weight of the arm is supported elsewhere, e.g., when the elbows are resting on a tabletop or arms of a chair.

Chronic contraction of muscles such as these can sometimes lead to tendinitis (inflammation of the tendons). To combat this, we need to teach the muscles to relax, and to alternate between relaxation and contraction.

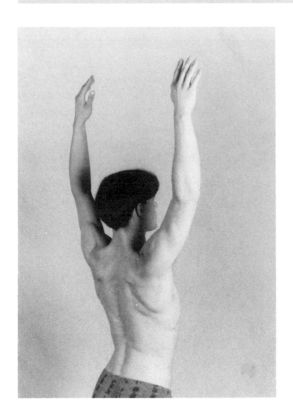

Superficial muscles

Latissimus dorsi originates from the spinous processes of T7-T12, the thoracolumbar fascia, and the sacral and iliac crests (see *AOM*, p. 125). It inserts anteriorly on the upper humerus. Shortening of this muscle may limit ROM of arm flexion. In this case, raising of the arms will provoke increased lordosis of the lumbar region and sometimes even anteversion of the pelvis. This is most noticeable when hanging by the arms from a bar. Stretching of this muscle loosens or frees joints in both the shoulder and lumbar/sacral areas.

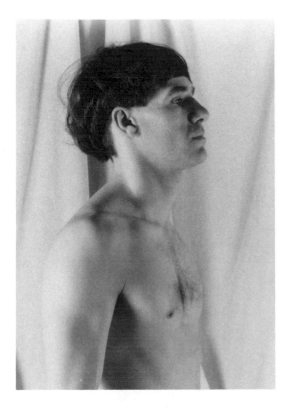

The **upper trapezius** originates from the occipital bone and cervical vertebrae, and inserts on the lateral clavicle and several points on the scapula (see *AOM*, p. 118). Symmetrical shortening of this muscle causes hyperextension of the head, often combined with anterior projection of the neck (caused by the sternocleidomastoid muscle), or with elevation of the shoulders. When all of these occur, the head seems to sink between the shoulders. Asymmetrical (one-sided) shortening of the upper trapezius has three possible results, which may occur in combination:
- extension and ipsilateral sidebending of the head
- ipsilateral sidebending of the cervical spine
- ipsilateral elevation of the shoulder girdle.

Exercises aimed at stretching this muscle can improve the movements and posture of the head, neck, and shoulders. However, such exercises must be done with care since they may also stretch the brachial plexus, an important nerve plexus which exits between the cervical vertebrae.

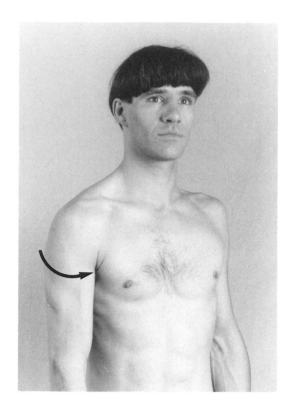

Pectoralis major originates from the clavicle, sternum, and costal cartilages 1–6, and inserts on the anterosuperior humerus (see *AOM*, p. 124). There is some mingling of aponeurotic fibers from the right and left portions of this muscle across the sternum. Contraction of this muscle on one side produces medial rotation and adduction of the humerus. Bilateral contraction leads to protraction of the shoulder girdle.

Pectoralis minor originates from ribs 3–5 anteriorly, runs almost straight upward, and inserts on the coracoid process of the scapula (see *AOM*, p. 116). Contraction of this muscle pulls the scapula forward and downward.

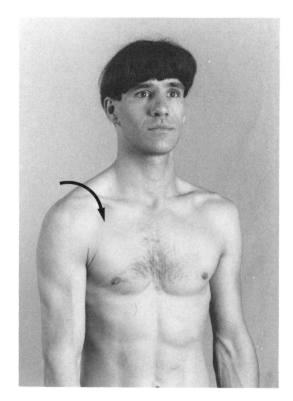

If pectoralis major and minor are shortened chronically and bilaterally, we observe that the shoulder joint (in side view) is held farther forward and downward than usual. To compensate for this, the thoracic spine is more rounded, and the cervical spine is extended in order to keep the head level. The upper trapezius and rhomboid muscles have an increased workload. Our first priority in this situation is to stretch the pectoral muscles.

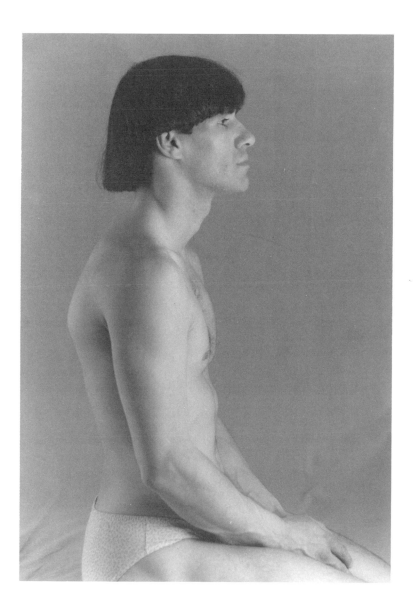

Strengthening of shoulder muscles

In daily life, demands for muscular strength of the shoulder are relatively low. In contrast to the legs, the arms are not routinely required to bear heavy loads. However, two points should be kept in mind:

- The rotator cuff muscles, as explained above, must remain in a state of partial contraction most of the time to support the weight of the arms. The strength of these muscles must be maintained, but they must also be able to relax when the opportunity arises.
- Occasional situations require greater-than-usual strength by the arm and shoulder: lifting a heavy external object, doing push-ups, hanging from a bar.

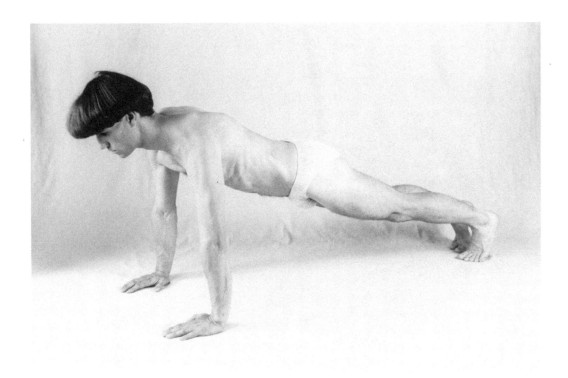

Our general goals in regard to the shoulder:

- Strengthen the superficial muscles, each one in accordance with the specific demands of our chosen physical discipline.
- Strengthen the deep muscles in similar fashion. In addition, train these muscles to relax when the weight of the arms is being supported by other means.
- When exercising shoulder muscles which also act on the neck (e.g., trapezius), make sure that the cervical vertebrae are correctly aligned.

Coordination of shoulder muscles

As mentioned at the beginning of the chapter, this is our primary concern in designing an exercise program for the shoulder. Ideally, we would like to be able to:

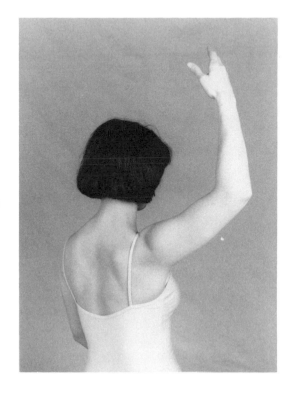

- move the scapula independently of the arm

- move the arm independently of the scapula

- differentiate one joint from the other when doing a movement which involves the whole shoulder girdle

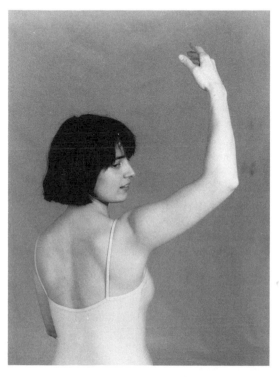

- move the neck independently of the shoulder girdle

- move the shoulder girdle independently of the neck

- differentiate specific joints or muscles when doing a movement which involves both the neck and shoulder girdle.

Fixing the scapula

By "fixing" we mean holding the scapula in place so that it serves as a stable anchoring point for muscles moving the arm. Fixing of any bone generally means simultaneous contraction of two major opposing muscles. In the case of the scapula, this means the middle trapezius and serratus anterior (see *AOM*, p. 115).

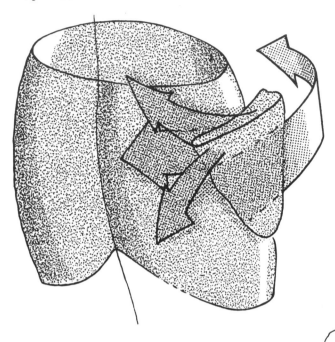

If the superior portion of the trapezius (instead of the middle one) is contracted in an attempt to fix the scapula, the entire shoulder girdle will rotate upward when the arm is raised to lift a heavy weight.

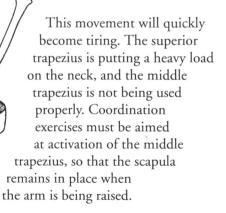

This movement will quickly become tiring. The superior trapezius is putting a heavy load on the neck, and the middle trapezius is not being used properly. Coordination exercises must be aimed at activation of the middle trapezius, so that the scapula remains in place when the arm is being raised.

Keeping the humeral head low when moving the arm

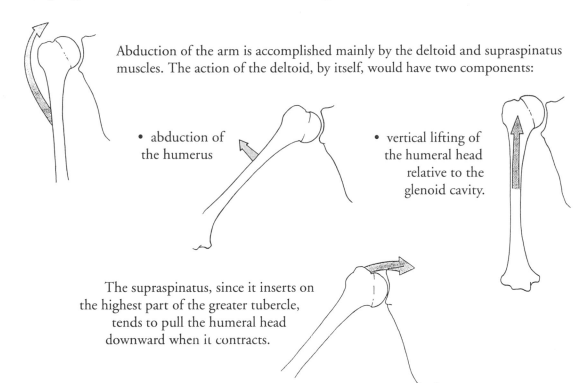

Abduction of the arm is accomplished mainly by the deltoid and supraspinatus muscles. The action of the deltoid, by itself, would have two components:

- abduction of the humerus

- vertical lifting of the humeral head relative to the glenoid cavity.

The supraspinatus, since it inserts on the highest part of the greater tubercle, tends to pull the humeral head downward when it contracts.

However, the deltoid is a much larger muscle and its action tends to dominate, i.e., during abduction of the arm the humeral head is typically pushed upward. There is a **coracoacromial ligament** which spans over the top of the shoulder joint like a bridge.

During repeated upward movement of the humeral head, the horizontal external border of this ligament may rub against and irritate the tendon of the supraspinatus. To a lesser extent, the same thing can happen to other rotator cuff muscles during abduction combined with flexion or extension.

You can see the importance of exercises aimed at keeping the humeral head low while raising the arm (see pp. 112–13).

Practice pages: Shoulder

Stretching the shoulder joint

For subjects with extremely restricted shoulder ROM, especially involving pain, physiotherapy may be most appropriate. However, the following movements, if they can be performed without pain, are often helpful in reducing stiffness.

ANTERIOR MOVEMENT

Start by practicing this in discrete steps, then combine them into a smooth flowing movement.

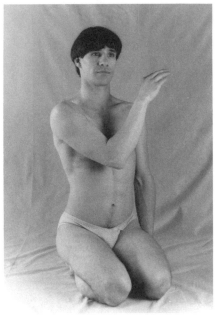

Adduct the arm in front of the body, elbow roughly next to the navel. Bend the elbow. Hand is near the opposite shoulder, shoulder joint is still adducted and slightly medially rotated.

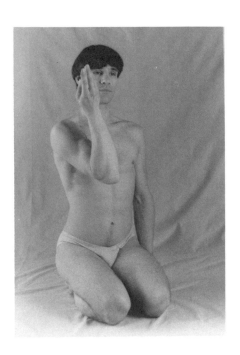

Abduct and laterally rotate shoulder joint. Hand is in the same sagittal plane as the shoulder joint, at the level of the face.

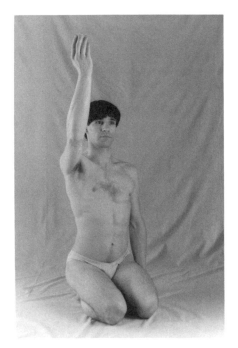

Move hand upward. Shoulder is flexed, elbow is extended.

Return to starting position.

In this example, the left hand could be used to guide the right hand if necessary.

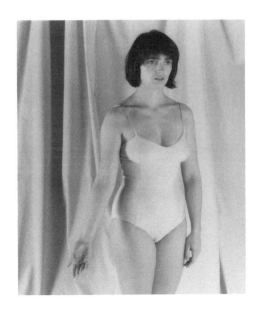

LATERAL MOVEMENT

Start with arm hanging relaxed at side.

Laterally rotate arm
(the right arm in this
example) as far as possible.

Abduct the arm, while
maintaining lateral
rotation. Do not force
the movement.

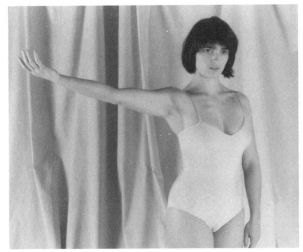

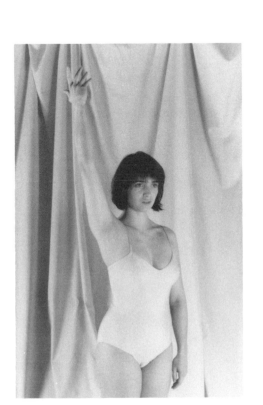

Continue abduction until
the arm is pointing up,
or as high as possible.
Look for the "passage"
so that the arm goes up
without any stiffness
or pain.

Return to starting position and repeat.

If this sequence is practiced and turned into a
flowing movement, it can restore the ability to
raise the arm even when stiffness has prevented
it from doing so for a long time.

Global articular and muscular stretching

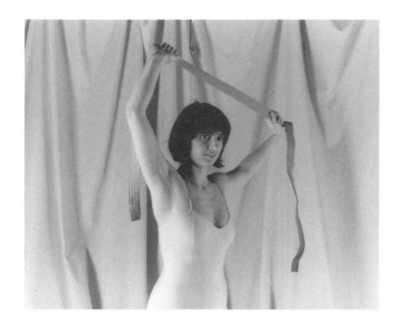

In either a standing
or sitting position,
hold a belt or stick
with both hands.

Alternating from side
to side, pull down
(adduct) with one
arm such that the
other arm is passively
pulled against the head.

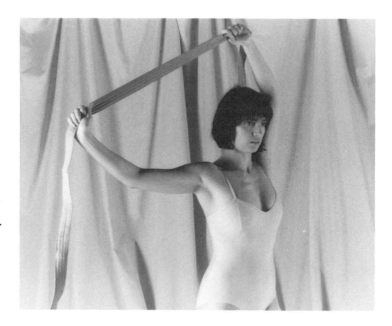

The only muscular action on the passive side is the grasping of the belt by the hand.
During this exercise, you can progressively try to lower the shoulder girdle or the humeral
head (see pp. 112–13).

Swaying and dangling movements

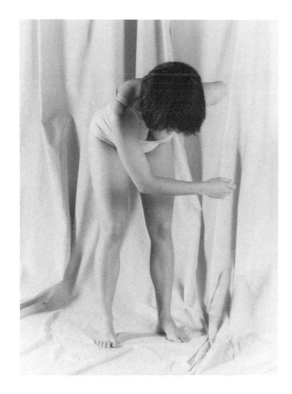

Lean forward from a standing position. Hips, knees, and trunk are all partly flexed. The trunk can also be bent to one side or the other. Swing the arms (one at a time) in many different directions: circles, figure eights, diagonal movements, etc.

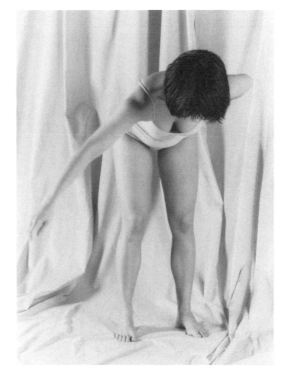

The rotator cuff and other muscles are partly contracted to support the weight of the arm. The benefit of this exercise is that it teaches fluidity of movement in combination with muscle tonus.

Stretching the shoulder muscles

STRETCHING THE LATISSIMUS DORSI

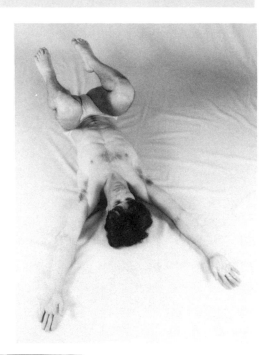

Lie on the back with hips flexed and knees near the chest. This position causes retroversion of the pelvis and reduces lordosis in the lumbar spine.

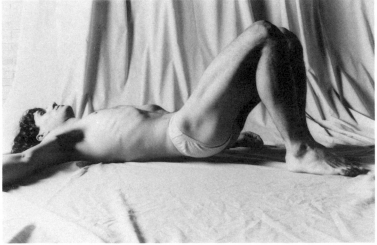

Alternatively, retrovert the pelvis by lifting, plant the feet on the mat and use muscular contractions of the leg muscles to pull the sacrum toward the feet.

Then, stretch and flatten the cervical spine by flexing the head, or pressing C4 against the floor. Place the hands on either side of the head. The spine should now be well stretched out posteriorly. Inhale deeply so as to lower the rib cage and press the back against the floor.

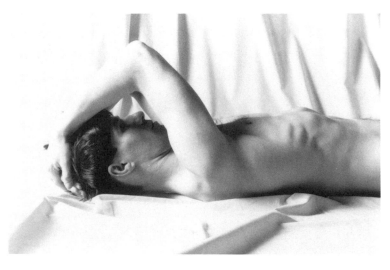

STRETCHING THE TRAPEZIUS

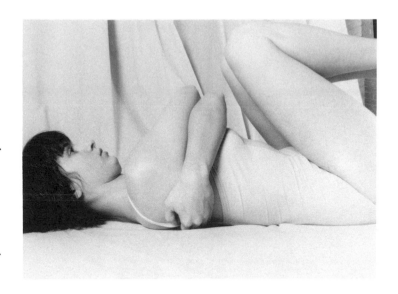

Lie on the back, hips flexed, knees near the chest so that the pelvis is retroverted and the lumbar arch flattened as above. Flatten the cervical spine as above. This tends to raise the thoracic spine off the floor. Flatten it as well by crossing both arms over the chest and around the ribs.

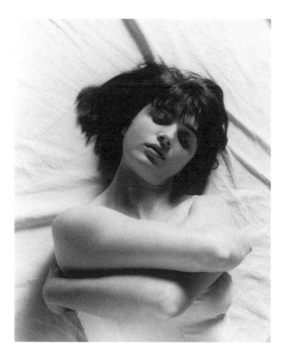

See if you can grab the lateral edges of the scapulas to pull them even further apart. While keeping the neck flattened, tilt the head to one side.

You will feel a stretching sensation on the opposite side of the neck. Never go so far that you provoke pinching or burning sensations. Slide the arm and hand down the body on the side of the stretch. Rotate the head slightly to one side and the other. You will feel stretching of different bundles of the superior trapezius.

STRETCHING THE PECTORALIS MAJOR

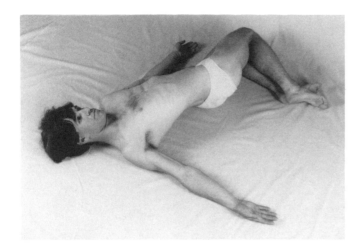

For the right pectoralis major:
Lie down on the left side,
flexing the legs and moving
them around to achieve balance
and stability. Abduct the
right arm as shown.

Rotate the torso to the right until
the elbow and forearm are in
contact with the floor, but keep
the shoulder off the floor. This
will require a twisting movement
at the waist. (It is not the amount
of twisting that matters, but that
the twisting leaves the shoulder at
the right height. The range of the
twisting movement may therefore
vary from one person to the next.)

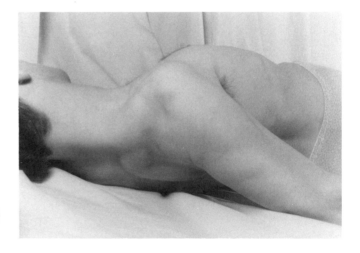

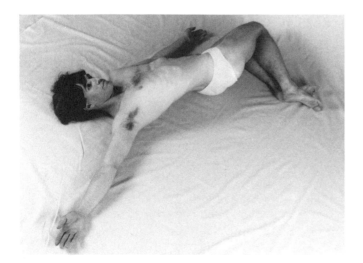

Next, make the hand traverse
the arc of a circle by circumducting the shoulder. At some
point, you should feel the
stretching of the pectoralis
major distal to the shoulder.

A burning or pinching sensation
means you are stretching too
much, and should lower the
shoulder closer to the floor.

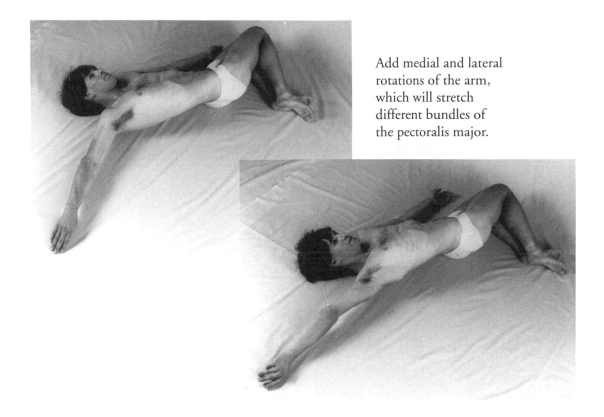

Add medial and lateral rotations of the arm, which will stretch different bundles of the pectoralis major.

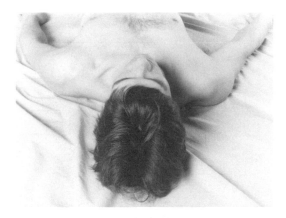

After this exercise, lie flat on your back with the arms along the sides. You should notice a difference between the two shoulders.

On the non-stretched side: The medial border of the scapula is more closely pressed against the floor than is the lateral border. The upper arm does not touch the floor. The humerus is medially rotated. The deltoid and pectoralis major are separated by a visible groove.

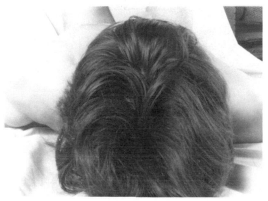

On the stretched side: The scapula rests flat on the floor. The upper arm touches the floor. The humerus is in neutral rotation. The deltoid and pectoralis major form an almost continuous muscular sheet.

STRETCHING THE PECTORALIS MINOR

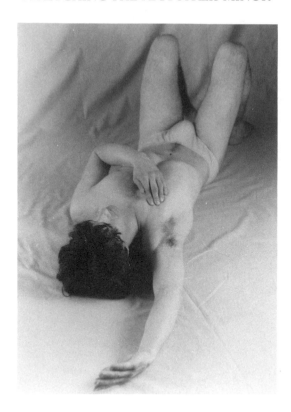

Lie flat on the back. Flex the arm above the head, hand resting on the floor.

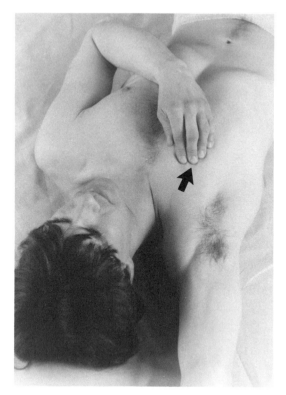

Exhale fully, so that the ribs are lowered toward the floor. You can use the free hand to press the sternum or ribs downward.

Note: For people with very stiff shoulders (e.g., those unable to place the arms on the floor above the head), exercises for the pectoralis major or minor should be done gradually, perhaps with the help of a partner moving the arm.

Strengthening the shoulder muscles

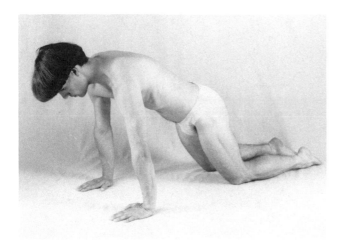

ANTERIOR MUSCLES

Start in a push-up position, knees on the floor, most of the weight on the hands.

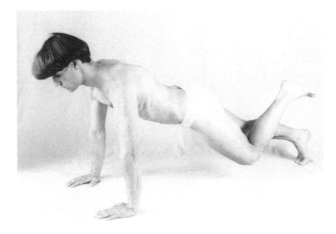

All the shoulder muscles are contracting, particularly the anterior ones: pectoralis major and minor, and the anterior deltoid. To increase the load on these muscles, lift the knees off the ground and then put one foot in the air.

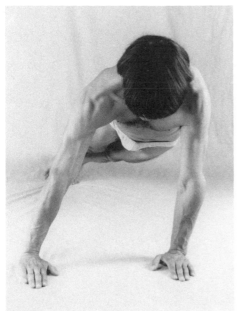

Next, put all the weight on one hand while resting the other, and vice versa.

SERRATUS ANTERIOR

Normally, in a hands/knees position, the lordosis of the thoracic spine tends to flatten out and the sternum comes closer to the floor. Consciously counteract this by arching the thoracic spine. The scapulas will move apart slightly, and their medial borders will be flattened.

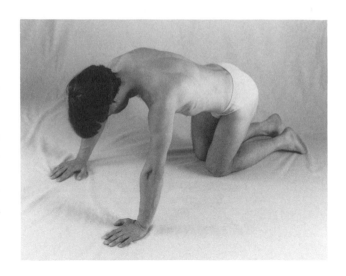

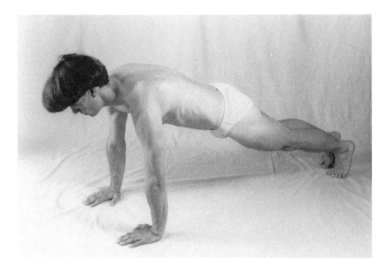

To better appreciate this movement, try doing it on one side at a time. For more intense strengthening of the serratus, follow the same exercise as described above for the anterior muscles.

To isolate the movement of the scapula: Retract the scapulas by clasping the hands behind the back as shown. The medial borders of the scapulas will project away from the ribcage. Return the arms forward and feel the medial scapular borders move closer to the ribs. Try to feel the sensations of the serratus anterior under the scapula and on the lateral ribcage.

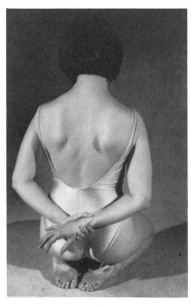

POSTERIOR MUSCLES

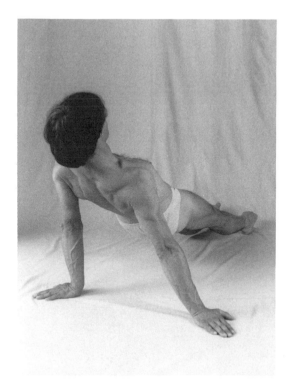

Support the body off the ground with the hands, face up, trunk and legs straight.

The posterior shoulder muscles are working hard in this position: rhomboids, trapezius, posterior deltoids. The head may be flexed forward, or held back (the latter position will make the anterior neck muscles work harder).

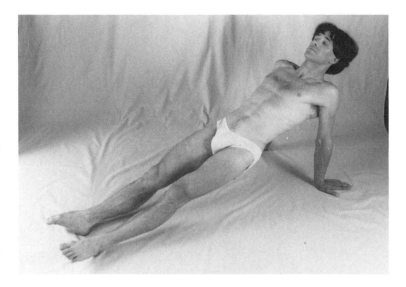

The triceps are also contracting strongly here to keep the elbows extended. In these situations of intense muscular activity, it is important to practice some of the coordination exercises described on the next few pages.

Coordination of shoulder muscles

COORDINATION OF SHOULDERS AND NECK

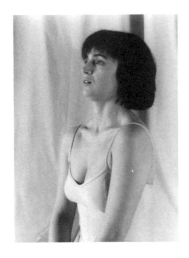

Flex the shoulder girdle (move it forward). This will protract the scapulas at the back.

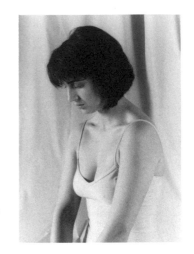

While maintaining this position, move the head and neck in various directions: flexion,

left and right rotation,

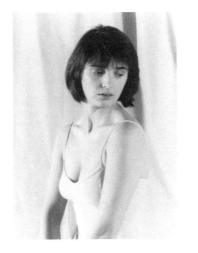

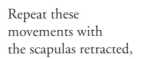

and sidebending (not shown).

Repeat these movements with the scapulas retracted,

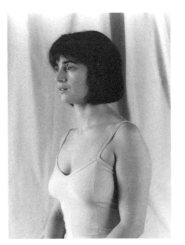

and in neutral position. This will increase your awareness of the different muscle activities and improve their coordination.

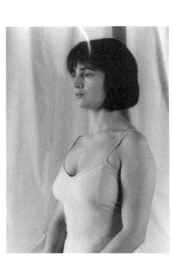

ACTIVE LOWERING OF THE SCAPULA

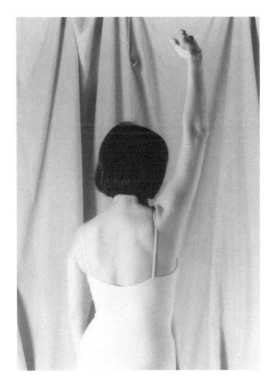

Flex or abduct your arm above
the head. Let the scapula move
strongly in upward rotation, with
its inferior angle moving away
from the midline.

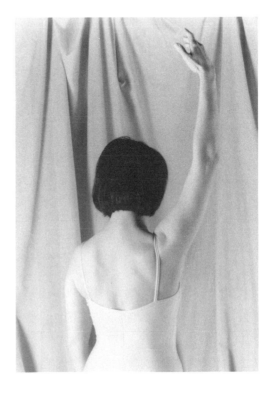

With the arm still raised, try consciously
to lower (depress) the scapula. You should
feel the superior trapezius relax and the
entire shoulder girdle move down.

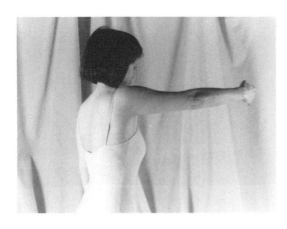

Next, flex the shoulder
so the arm is pointing forward.

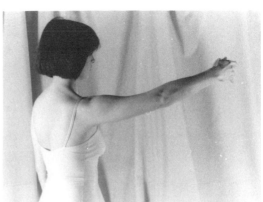

Consciously pull the
scapula posteriorly (retract).

Alternate between the arm-up and arm-front positions, trying to keep the scapula down and back.

LOWERING THE HUMERAL HEAD

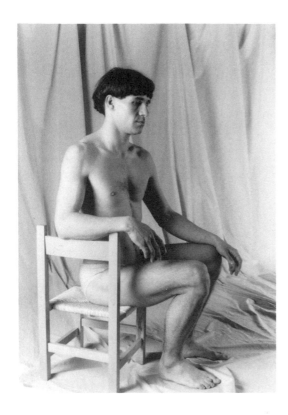

Sit down with a support
for the elbow (ideally,
the arm of a chair).

Focus your mind on the feeling
that the elbow is being supported
externally, and that the superior
trapezius is being released from
its usual job of supporting
the weight of the arm.

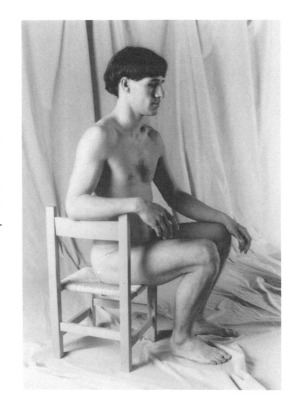

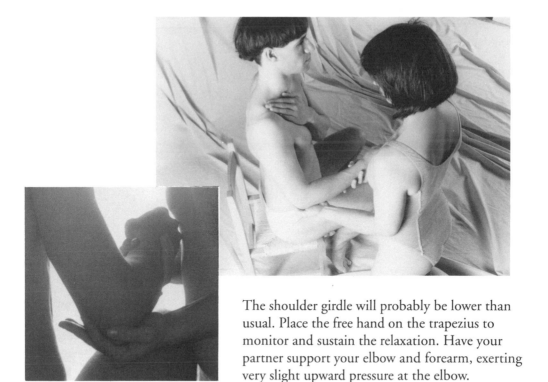

The shoulder girdle will probably be lower than usual. Place the free hand on the trapezius to monitor and sustain the relaxation. Have your partner support your elbow and forearm, exerting very slight upward pressure at the elbow.

This pushes the humerus upward against the deltoid. Oppose this movement by actively lowering not the shoulder girdle, but the humeral head away from the acromion process of the scapula. You will feel the sensation lower down. A dimple-like depression will appear in the deltoid muscle, just lateral to the protrusion of the acromion.

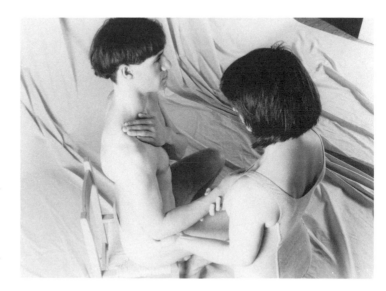

Finally, try to flex the arm, with initially small but progressively larger ROM, while keeping the humeral head lowered.

CHAPTER FOUR

The Elbow & Forearm

There are two bones in the forearm: the **ulna** and the **radius**. The elbow joint, where the distal humerus articulates with the proximal ulna, is a hinge joint allowing only flexion and extension. The radius can cross over the ulna in the movement called pronation. These movements, combined with movements at the shoulder and wrist joints, allow us to place the hand in almost any desired position and orientation.

Movements

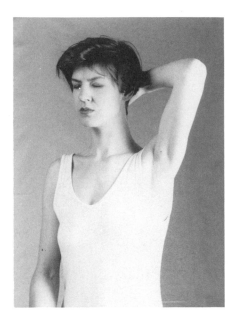

In **flexion** of the elbow, the anterior surfaces of the arm and forearm move closer to each other.

This movement is involved in bringing the hand to the mouth, behind the head, etc.

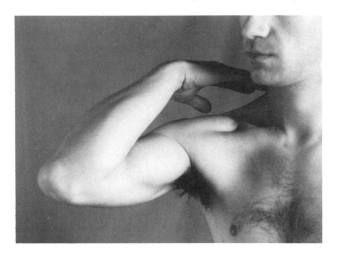

In **extension** of the elbow, the anterior surfaces of the arm and forearm move away from each other until they are aligned (i.e., in anatomical position).

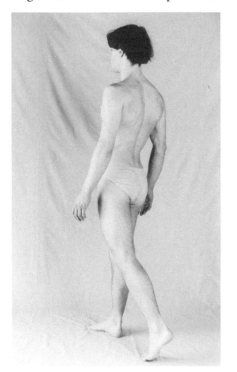

Increase of the angle beyond 180° is usually impossible, because the olecranon process of the ulna contacts the corresponding fossa of the humerus (see *AOM*, pp. 133–34).

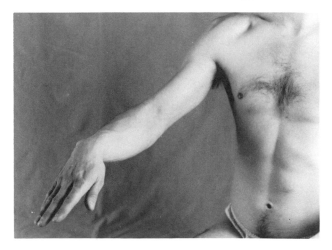

Loss of ability to flex or extend the elbow is rare. When it occurs, it interferes with nearly all the normal activities of human life (eating, dressing, writing, driving, etc.)

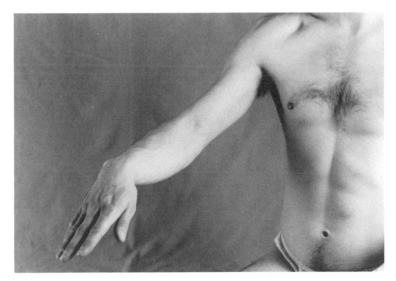

In **pronation**, the radius crosses over the ulna such that the palm of the hand faces posteriorly and the thumb is medial.

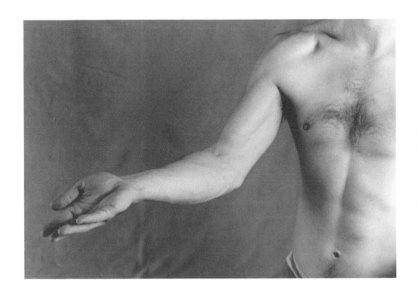

In **supination**, the radius returns to anatomical position and becomes parallel to the ulna, the palm faces anteriorly, and the thumb is lateral.

These movements are essential in a variety of twisting activities such as opening a jar or turning a doorknob.

Flexibility

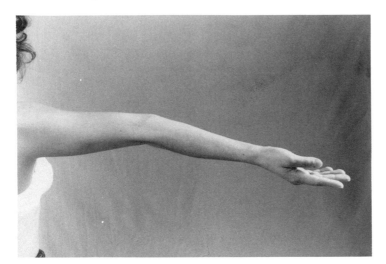

Elbow extension normally does not go past 180°, as noted above. The exception, called **recurvatum**, is due to abnormal shape of the bone surfaces.

This condition causes stress when heavy loads are applied to the elbow. In this case, elbow flexors (mainly brachialis and biceps brachii) must be contracted more than usual to oppose the hyperextension at the joint.

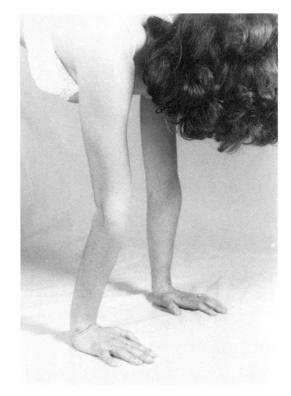

Rotation at the elbow joint is prevented by ligaments and by the shape of the articulating surfaces, particularly the fitting of the olecranon process into its fossa when the elbow is extended.

The joint capsule of the elbow is comparatively loose posteriorly (to facilitate flexion), and more resistant anteriorly (to limit extension). Some very strong ligaments on either side of the joint prevent lateral or medial movements.

The fasciae of the muscles of the anterior arm and forearm are connected to the palmar aponeurosis of the hand (see *AOM*, p. 157) and to the fasciae of the shoulder muscles. Thus, there is a continuity of connective tissue structures from the fingers to the shoulders, and even to the opposite shoulder and arm (via the pectoralis major muscles whose fasciae meet at the sternum). Stretching exercises for the elbow muscles, therefore, are preferably done bilaterally and in conjunction with shoulder stretching.

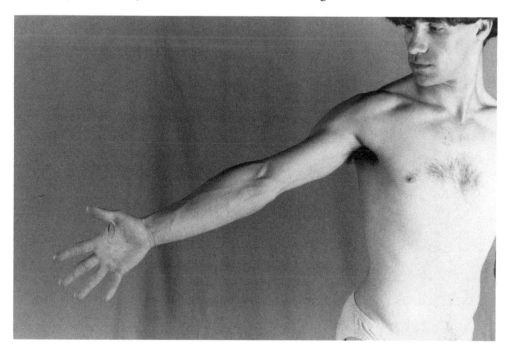

Pronation is limited by contact between the shafts of the radius and ulna. There is an **interosseous membrane** between the shafts of these two bones (see *AOM*, p. 143). Stiffening or inflammation of this membrane (typically felt as deep pain) can also restrict pronation and supination. Muscular braking action in pronation and supination is negligible.

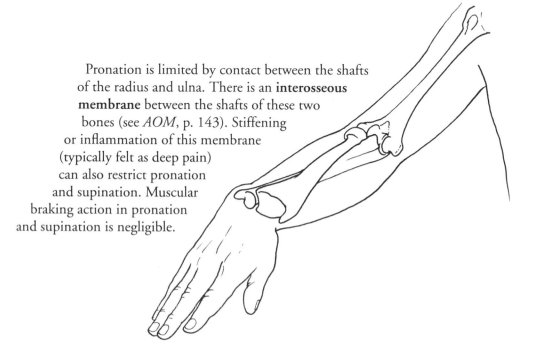

Muscular strength

The large muscles which cross the elbow anteriorly are brachialis, brachioradialis, biceps brachii, and pronator teres (see *AOM*, pp. 138–39 and 145). They are responsible for flexion and supination/pronation. There are also some small, localized epicondylar and epitrochlear muscles crossing the joint anteriorly. The only posterior muscles crossing the elbow, and the only extensors of the joint, are triceps brachii, which has one origin on the scapula and two origins on the humerus, and the much smaller anconeus (*AOM*, p. 140). We see a clear predominance of flexor over extensor muscles in terms of numbers and strength. This corresponds to the greater frequency of flexion movements in everyday life. The same trend can be observed for muscles moving the shoulder, wrist, and hand.

Strength of the elbow flexors and extensors can be maintained in two ways:

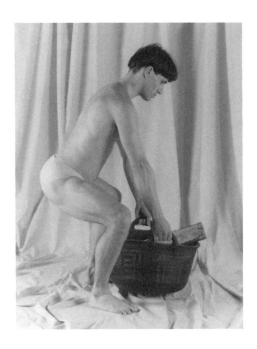

- through "open chain" exercises where the arms hold up some load

- through "closed chain" exercises where the body is partly or entirely supported by the arms.

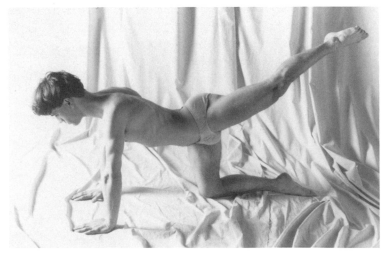

Supination is achieved by the biceps (long head), supinator (see *AOM*, p. 146), brachioradialis, and small epicondylar muscles. Pronation is achieved by pronator teres and pronator quadratus, brachioradialis, and small epitrochlear muscles. In terms of size and strength, supinators predominate over pronators.

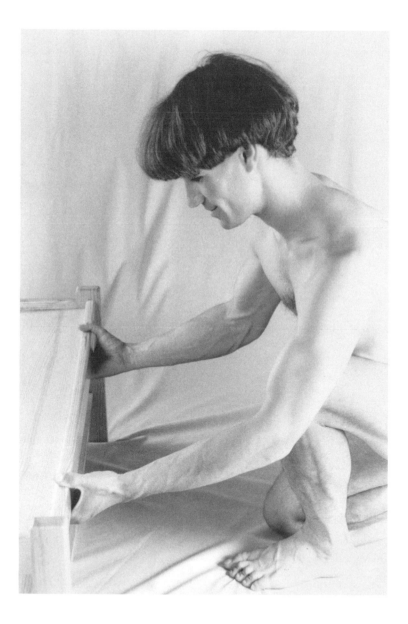

Since flexion and supination are "preferred" over extension and pronation, the most efficient position for lifting heavy objects is one where the elbow is slightly flexed and the forearm is supinated.

Coordination

For coordination of arm movements, we prefer to synchronize flexion/extension of the elbow, pronation/supination of the forearm, and the large movements of the shoulder joint. This leads to "diagonal" movements in which the arm crosses the body and the hand shifts its position. It can also be helpful to work on movements of the elbow and wrist independently of those of the shoulder, or vice versa.

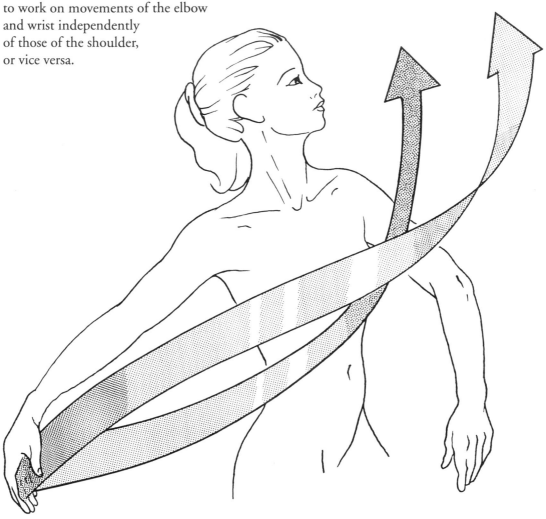

Practice pages for elbow and forearm exercises will be combined with those for the wrist and hand in the following chapter.

CHAPTER FIVE

The Wrist & Hand

In humans the primary functions of the feet remain the same as for our distant ancestors: locomotion and support. The musculature of the feet is adapted for these functions.

Our hands are an entirely different story. As humans have evolved, the hands have become capable of a huge variety of actions, ranging from the very forceful to the very delicate: swinging an axe, throwing a ball, peeling an orange, playing the piano, painting a model airplane, and so forth.

We cannot hope to describe all the possible complex movements of the hand, or specific exercises for each one. However, the practice pages in this chapter include some good general exercises for improving flexibility, strength, and coordination of the hands, in conjunction with the wrists and elbows.

Wrist movements

In **flexion** the angle between the palm of the hand and the anterior surface of the forearm decreases.

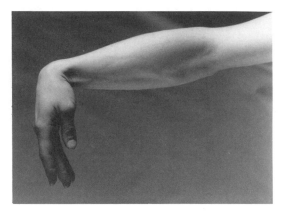

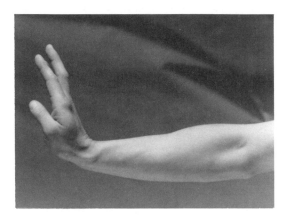

In **extension** the angle between the posterior hand and posterior forearm decreases. Normal ROM for both flexion and extension is around 85°–90°.

In **abduction** the angle formed by the lateral edges of the hand and forearm decreases, and the thumb moves closer to the radius.

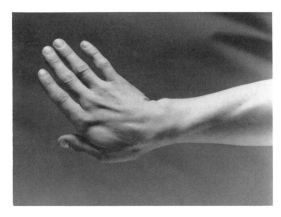

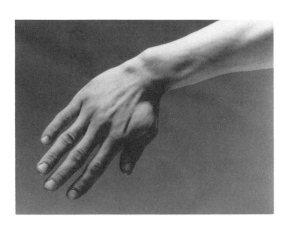

In **adduction** the angle formed by the medial edges of the hand and forearm decreases, and the thumb moves farther from the radius.

Almost no rotation is possible at the wrist joint. Students often confuse pronation/supination of the forearm with wrist rotation. By clamping your other hand firmly around the forearm and immobilizing the radius and ulna, you can see that the wrist does not rotate by itself. However, the hand can perform a kind of circumduction which really consists of combined flexion, extension, abduction, and adduction.

Functionally, loss of mobility at the wrist presents less of a handicap than loss of mobility at the elbow or at the radioulnar joints where pronation/supination occur.

Wrist flexibility

Extension of the wrist is restricted by contact between the scaphoid and lunate bones (*AOM*, p. 149) and the posterior border of the radius. Abduction and adduction are limited by contact between the carpal bones and the styloid processes of the radius and ulna (*AOM*, p. 133).

The joint capsule and ligaments of the wrist have minimal braking effect on wrist movements.

There are no muscles whose bodies pass over the wrist joint. Rather, the wrist is spanned by tendons of numerous muscles whose bodies are located in the forearm area and whose origins are on the radius, ulna, and/or humerus. Many of the muscles which insert on and move the fingers cross the elbow as well as the wrist joint.

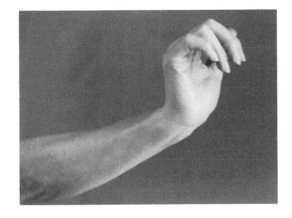

The reason that hyperextending the wrist causes flexion of the fingers is that the tendons of the flexor muscles are being pulled

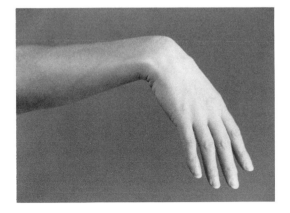

However, flexing the wrist does not cause extension of the fingers; the tendons of the extensor muscles have more "slack."

To regain flexibility in the flexor muscles, try stretching them with movements going all the way to the tips of the fingers, i.e., simultaneously hyperextend the wrist and pull the fingertips back.

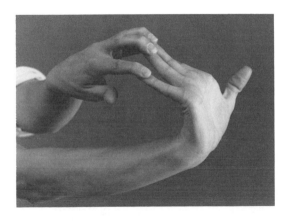

Wrist strength and coordination

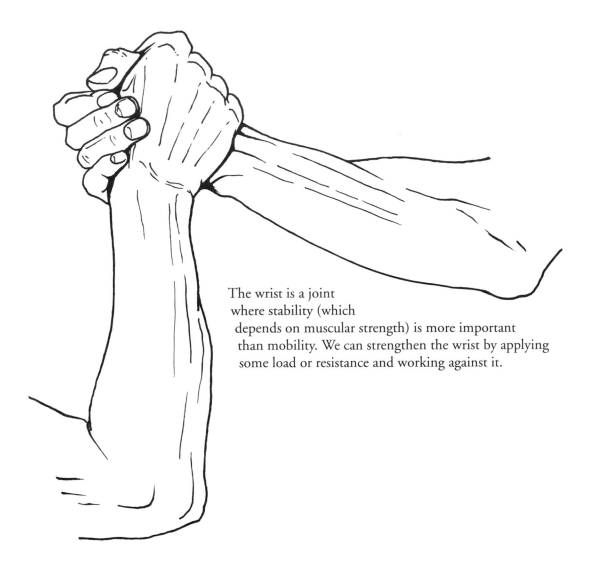

The wrist is a joint
where stability (which
depends on muscular strength) is more important
than mobility. We can strengthen the wrist by applying
some load or resistance and working against it.

The "preferred" position of the wrist when working against resistance is slightly extended and abducted, because of the shapes of the articular surfaces and the orientation of the tendons. In this same position the fingers have the most strength for flexion, because the flexor tendons are already taut.

Effective wrist coordination exercises go "diagonally" from this extension/abduction position to a flexion/adduction position. They can be combined with shoulder or elbow movements.

Hand/finger movements & flexibility

The **metacarpophalangeal joints** can undergo:

- flexion/extension

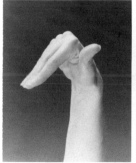
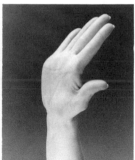

- abduction/adduction

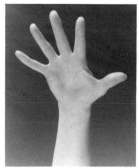
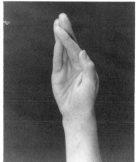

- slight rotation.

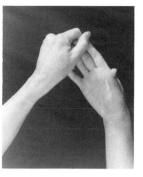

The **proximal interphalangeal joints** undergo flexion only.

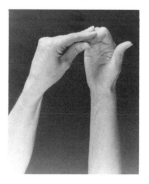

The **distal interphalangeal joints** undergo flexion and varying degrees of extension, which depends on the finger and the individual.

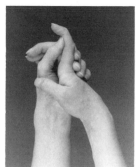
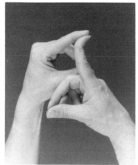

Limitation of these movements is due mostly to ligaments, not to the shape of articulating bony surfaces. As mentioned above, the muscles which insert on and move the fingers are polyarticular; they cross the wrist and often the elbow joint. They typically have very long tendons, and the muscle bodies are far away from the fingers. Therefore the ROM of the fingers will depend on the positions of the wrist and elbow.

Hand strength

There are intrinsic hand muscles originating from the carpals or metacarpals (see *AOM*, pp. 170–74), as well as the larger extrinsic hand muscles which cross the wrist joint (see *AOM*, pp. 166–70). In terms of strength, the finger flexors dominate the extensors. This reflects the importance of gripping and holding actions of the hand.

Hand coordination

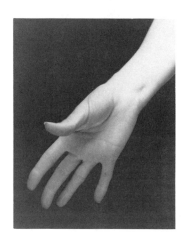

The three prominent folds on the palm are related to the most common coordinated finger movements. The "life line," closest to the thumb, results from the opposing movement in which the thumb moves toward the other fingers.

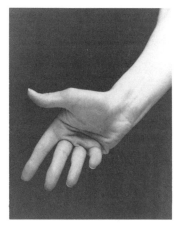

Flexion of metacarpophalangeals II–V makes a double fold since the four fingers don't move as a unit. Finger V (little finger) flexes earlier and with greater ROM than finger II (index finger).

For this reason, the palm tends to form a curved groove where any held object will fit snugly.

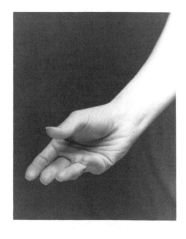

Practice pages: Elbow, wrist & hand

General stretching

Sit on your heels. Extend the shoulder joints as far back as possible. At the same time, keep the elbows, wrists, and finger joints extended. Abduct (spread apart) the fingers.

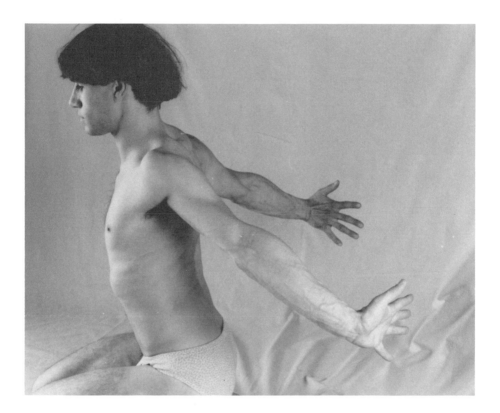

If some fingers spread apart less easily than others, work on those. Concentrate on extending all the phalanges of each finger. You can do this exercise one arm at a time, then both together. It is normal to have a pronounced depression between the shoulder blades. If you have a partner, he or she can help by gently pressing the arms and hands even farther back.

This exercise stretches all the aponeuroses and flexor muscles of the upper limbs, from the sternum to the fingertips. *Note:* This exercise puts the head of the humerus in an unstable position. If you have had a sprain or dislocation of the shoulder (especially if more than once), avoid this exercise.

Strengthening exercises

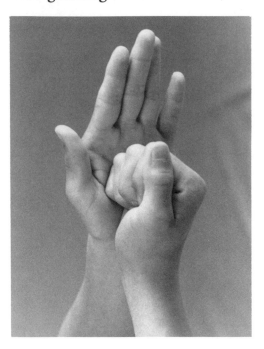

Make a fist with the right hand. With the left hand, apply pressure first to the medial border,

then the lateral border of the right hand.

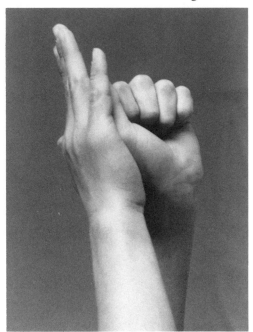

This strengthens the wrist flexors of the left hand, and the wrist and finger adductors of the right hand. Repeat with the hands reversed.

Extend the fingers of the right hand, and press against the back of the right hand with the left. This works the wrist and finger extensors.

Press both hands together with the wrists hyper-extended. This will develop strength and stability in the wrists.

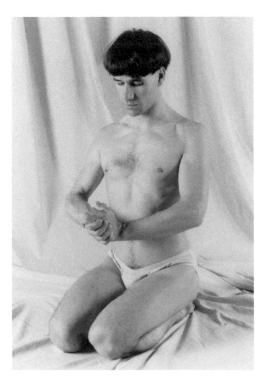

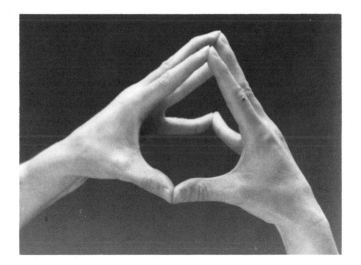

Keep the fingers straight and place the fingertips together. Press strongly with both hands. This strengthens most of the flexors of the hands and arms, including pectoralis major.

Kneel and place the extended fingers of both hands against the floor. Put most of your upper body weight onto these fingers.

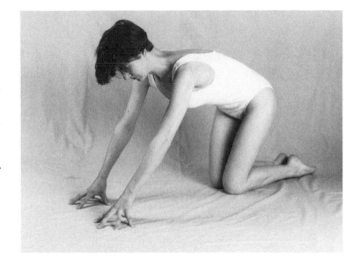

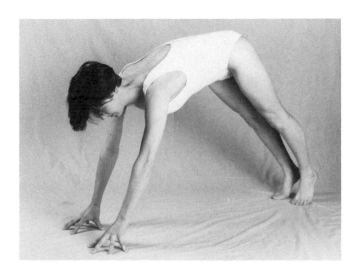

From the above position, raise the knees off the floor and straighten the legs. This increases the load on the fingers.

Coordination exercises

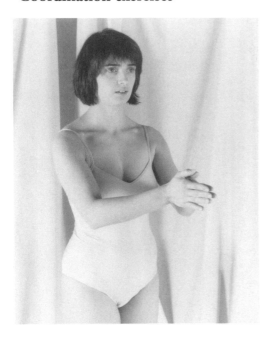

Stand up. Place your hands together in front of you, elbows partly flexed.

Keep the hands in the same place, but elevate the elbows and arms.

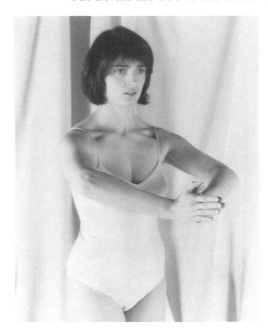

The elbows move apart from each other. Now move the elbows and arms downward, still keeping the hands in the same place. Work on maintaining continuity as you repeat these movements.

Do a similar sequence of movements but with the hands held 10 or 12 inches apart. Imagine you are holding an invisible ball between the hands. Again, try to keep the hands in the same place and concentrate on the continuity of the elbow and arm movements. Feel how you can initiate and guide the movement either from the shoulder (the abduction of the shoulder taking along the elbow and wrist), or from the hand (the "fixed" hand provides a pivot for movement of the forearm, which takes the arm with it).

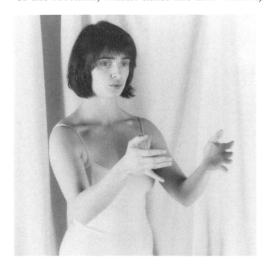

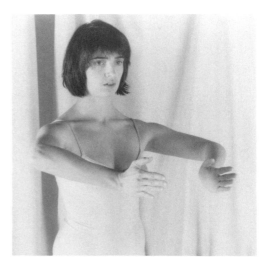

Perform a similar sequence, but with the elbows almost fully extended and hands together again.

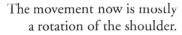

The movement now is mostly a rotation of the shoulder.

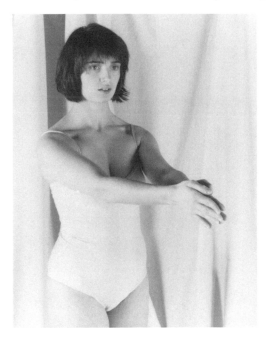

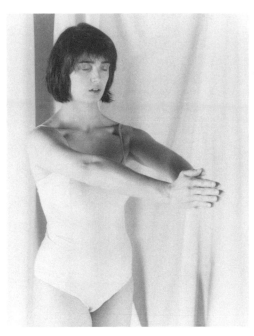

Continue, now with the hands held apart. Notice again how either the hands or shoulders can be visualized as the reference points for the movement.

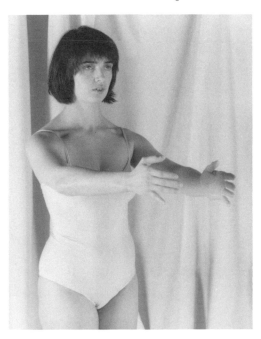

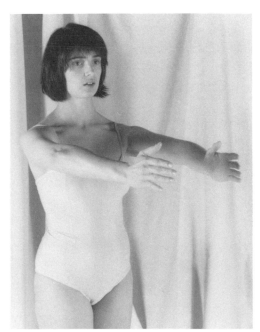

Experiment with different elbow angles and hand positions in this exercise.

Thinking about this "dual guiding" action helps us link the distal gestures of the hand to the shoulder (or even the trunk) and, conversely, to let the movements of the shoulder continue all the way to the hand.

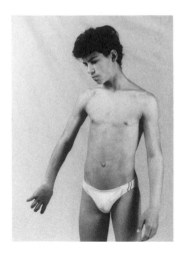

Another coordination exercise: Place one arm in
slight abduction, extension, and medial rotation.

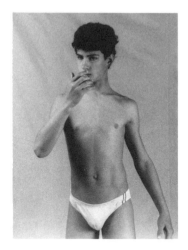
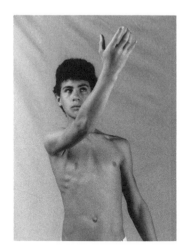

Move the arm diagonally upward and across the body,
with supination of the forearm bones. Reverse this
movement, so the arm ends up back where it started.

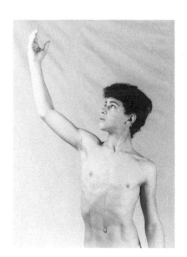

Now, start with the arm raised, abducted,
and laterally rotated, and the forearm supinated.

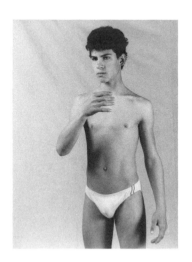
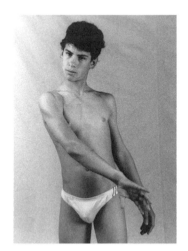

Move the arm diagonally downward and across the
body, with medial rotation of the shoulder and
pronation of the forearm.

Pass smoothly from the first of these large diagonal movements to the other, and back again, as
if drawing a giant figure eight in the air. Repeat with the other arm.

Another coordination exercise: Move the hand as if drawing a circle (clockwise direction) on an invisible wall in front of you. Start with a small circle, then make it progressively larger (continuous spiral movement of the hand). Repeat, this time with a counterclockwise direction.

Perform a similar exercise, but this time draw circles on an imaginary horizontal tabletop instead of a vertical wall. This is a more natural movement for the shoulder joint.

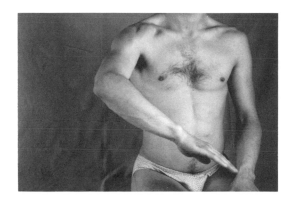

Repeat with vertical and horizontal figure eights instead of circles. Try making the eights oblique, e.g., have the upper loop of the eight come closer to the body, and the lower loop move farther away.

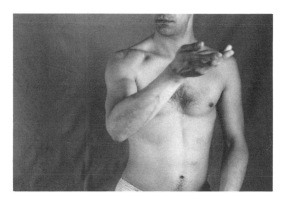

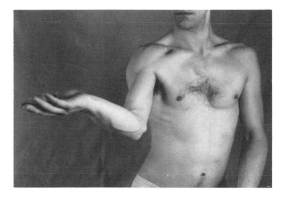

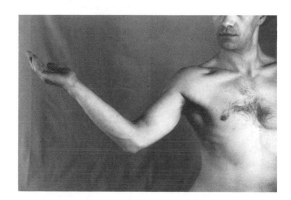

Finger exercises

These are just a few simple examples. You can think of many variations.

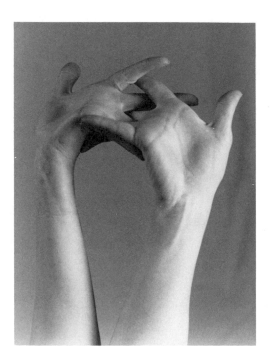

For general limbering and stretching of the hands, interlace all the fingers together with the palms facing the body at stomach level. Move the hands toward the head, turning the wrists so the palms are facing upward. Try to move the elbows closer together while keeping the fingers as interlaced as possible.

For coordination, try flexing the fingers in different ways, e.g., flex fingers II and V while leaving III and IV extended, or vice versa.

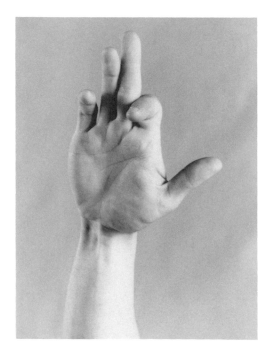

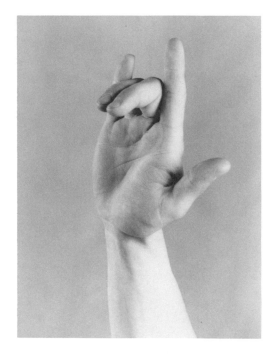

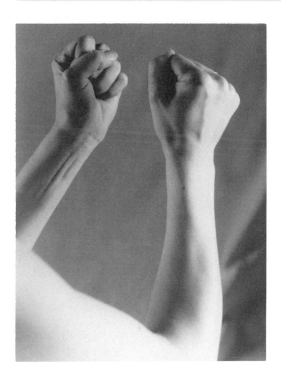

Start with closed fists.

Extend the fingers one by one:
thumb, index finger,

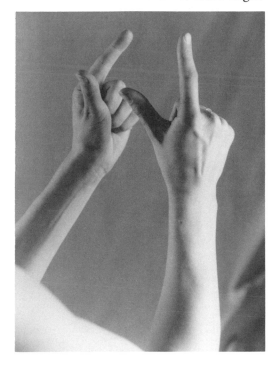

middle finger,

ring finger, little finger.

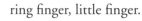

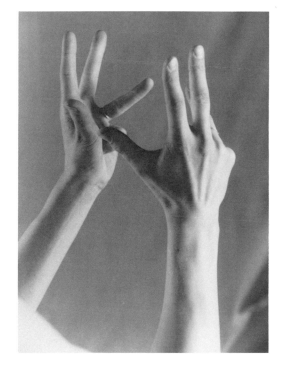

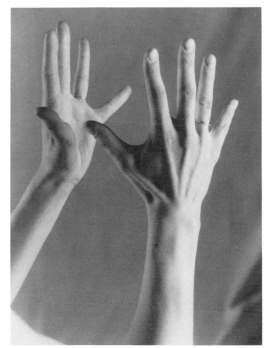

Repeat, but starting with the little finger and ending with the thumb.

Start with extended fingers and "close" them one at a time. Experiment with different orders.

CHAPTER SIX

The Hip

The pelvic girdle articulates above with the sacrum, and below with the two femurs. The hip joints, where the femoral heads form ball-and-socket joints with the acetabula (see *AOM*, pp. 180–81), constitute the intersection between the legs and the trunk. Stiffness at the hip joints will have adverse effects on the spine, the knee, and the foot. Such stiffness is quite rare in children, but fairly common in adults, especially with increasing age. Through proper exercise we can maintain ease of movement in the hip joint, and prevent or reduce stiffness.

Movements

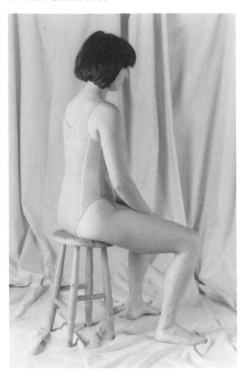

For the hip joint, we can refer to "femoral movement" (when the pelvis is fixed) or "pelvic movement" (when the femur is fixed).

In **femoral flexion** the anterior surface of the thigh moves closer to the anterior trunk. Examples from everyday life are walking, climbing stairs, and sitting down. Examples in ballet are forward leg movements and the plié.

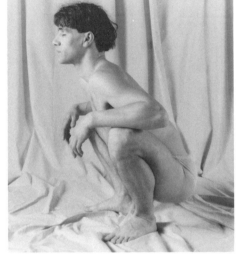

Flexion is often combined with other movements: with abduction in a sitting position with knees apart or in a squatting position;

with lateral rotation in pliés with the feet turned out.

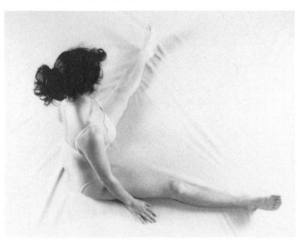

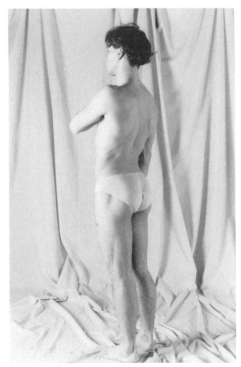

In **pelvic flexion**, or anteversion, the femur is fixed and the pelvis tilts forward. This movement is often confused with lumbar lordosis, even though it takes place at a different level (see p. 34).

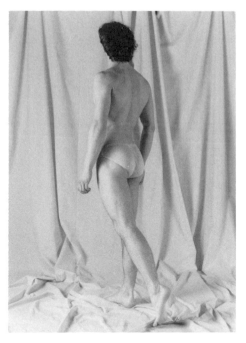

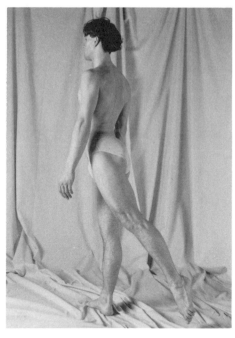

Femoral extension takes the posterior surface of the thigh closer to the back. We find it at certain points in walking or running.

The arabesque technique of classical ballet combines extension with lateral rotation.

ROM for hip extension is quite limited. Extension tends to induce anteversion of the pelvis, especially when combined with ipsilateral flexion of the knee. **Pelvic extension** or retroversion, where the femur is fixed and the pelvis tilts backward, is a movement often emphasized in dance classes where the instructor wishes to "erase the arching in the lower back" (see p. 32).

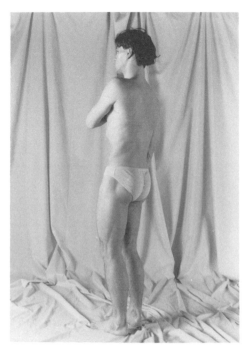

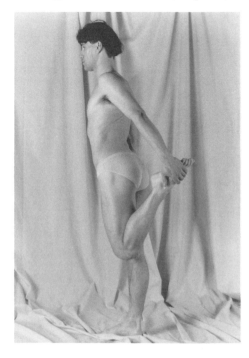

In **femoral abduction** the leg moves away from the midline, i.e., the angle between the lateral surface of the thigh and the trunk decreases.

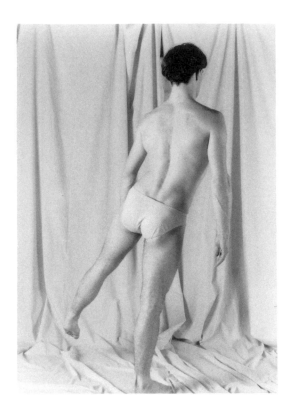

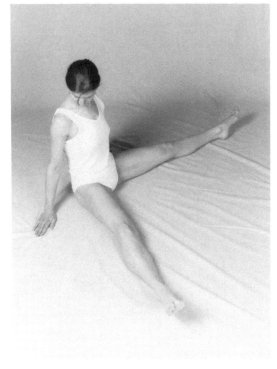

Abduction performed from anatomical position (with the knee facing forward) has limited ROM because the femoral neck hits the edge of the acetabulum. When abduction is combined with lateral rotation and flexion, ROM is much greater because the femur is in a different position (see *AOM*, p. 188).

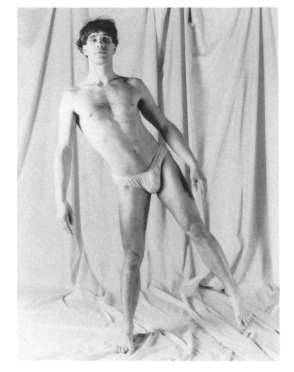

In **pelvic abduction** the pelvis tilts in a lateral direction relative to the fixed femur.

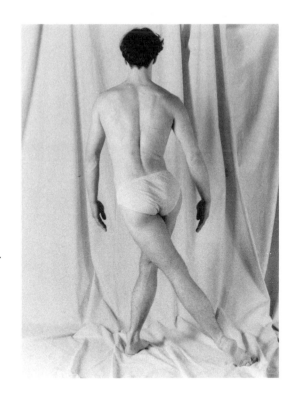

In **femoral adduction** the medial surface of the thigh moves toward or past the midline. When simply returning from an abducted position, adduction stops at the midline when one leg contacts the other. When combined with flexion or extension, as in the typical crossing movements of ballet, adduction can take the leg well past the midline.

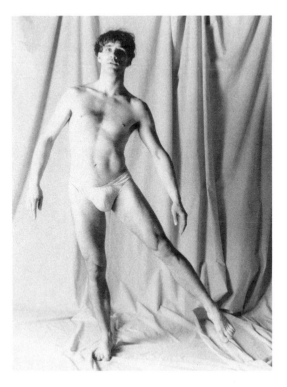

In **pelvic adduction** the pelvis tilts in a medial direction relative to the fixed femur.

The various pelvic movements mentioned above are common. Think about what's happening at your hip joints as you walk slowly, or shift your weight from one foot to the other in a standing position.

In rotations of the hip joint, the femur is turning on its own longitudinal axis like a screw driver. It is important to differentiate this from movements of the foot at the ankle joint. In **medial rotation** you will see the kneecap and foot moving medially.

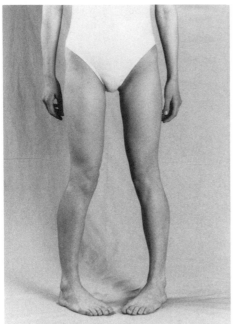

As usual, there is a corresponding movement where the femur is fixed and the pelvis rotates medially.

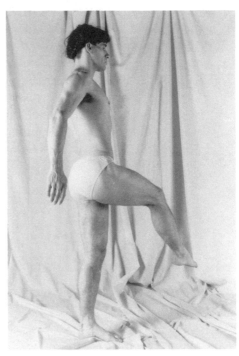

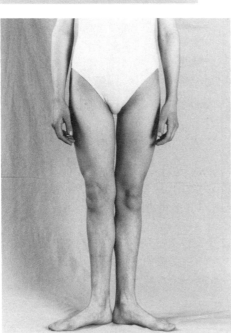

In **lateral rotation** the kneecap and foot move laterally. In classical ballet this is called "opening" and is often combined with other movements.

In the corresponding movement, the femur is fixed and the pelvis rotates laterally.

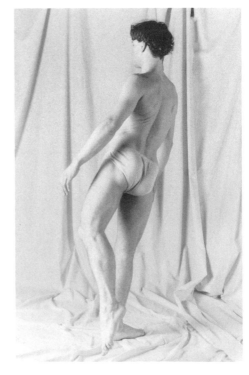

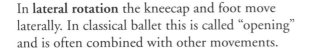

Movements of the pelvic bones

The ilium, ischium, and pubis are fused together at the acetabulum and no movement occurs between them here. However, slight movement is possible at the symphysis pubis and the

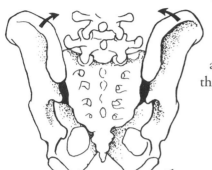

iliosacral joints. To feel some of these movements, try sitting on a stool with your weight on the ischial tuberosities ("sitting bones"). First, shift your weight onto one tuberosity and move the other one farther away before putting your weight onto it again. Here the symphysis pubis is put under stress at the bottom.

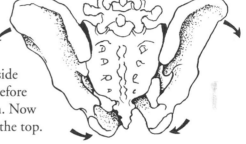

Then take the weight off one side and move the other side closer before distributing the weight evenly again. Now the symphysis is put under stress at the top.

Shift your weight onto one ischium and move the other one forward (or backward) before distributing your weight evenly

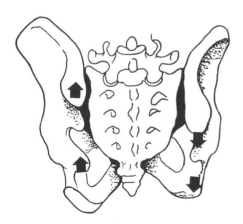

again. Now one ilium is in retroversion and the other in anteversion. The pubic symphysis is in torsion.

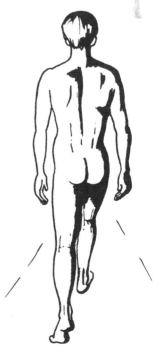

Movements of this type accompany virtually all movements at the hip joint. For instance, think about a person walking with long steps. On the side where the leg is stepping forward, the femur is in flexion and the ilium in retroversion. There are analogous pelvic bone movements which accompany extension, abduction, abduction, and rotation.

Flexibility of the hip

Good hip flexibility is important for many normal movements, and for simply feeling "at ease in one's body" during everyday life. As mentioned, however, stiffening at this joint is not uncommon in adults. What are the causes of this stiffening, and how can we prevent it?

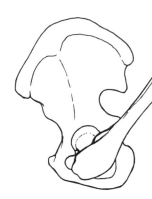

ROM at the hip is restricted by bony structures to a greater extent than ROM at the shoulder (see *AOM*, pp. 180–83). This restriction varies from one person to the next, and depends on early development.

The hip joint appears during the second month of fetal life. Like the rest of the skeleton, it starts out as cartilage. Ossification of the femoral head begins at a bony nucleus which appears around month five, and spreads toward the periphery. In the pelvis, three bony nuclei appear between months three to six, and spread out gradually to give rise to the ilium, ischium, and pubis. The Y-shaped intersection of these three bones forms the acetabulum. After birth, the acetabulum remains mostly cartilaginous for six months or so.

Bony nuclei of hip at one year of age

The outer surface of the femoral head and the inner surface of the acetabulum shape and mold each other during the first months of life. Each of these components depends on the presence of the other to ossify into the correct shape. The pressure of the femoral head should be directed mostly at the center of the Y-shaped intersection of the three pelvic bones.

The orientation of the hip can be tested at birth and some correction made if necessary. Often it is beneficial to wrap the legs in an abducted position. In some cultures and historical periods, babies have been tightly wrapped with the legs in adduction, which leads to improper orientation of the hip joints.

Pressure of the femoral head and acetabulum against each other result from resting position, from kicking and pushing movements, and (when the baby is old enough) from standing and walking. The "molding" process, combined with genetic factors, determines the exact shape of the articulating surfaces, the edge of the socket, and the neck of the femur. These bony shapes in turn determine the ROM, braking action, and stability of the hip joint (see *AOM*, pp. 182–83, 188–89).

Relative flexibility (or stiffness) of the hip joint varies widely among different people. If restrictions of ROM are directly related to bony structures, nothing can be done to change this, and there is no point in encouraging the individual to further limber up the area or to stretch beyond the imposed bony limits. We can, however, try to prevent harmful "compensations" from taking place in the vertebral joints, knee, etc.

How can you identify hip stiffness which originates in the bony structure? In a class situation, this is very difficult. One rule that may be helpful is that bone-related stiffness is often felt as blockage at the apex of the angle of movement, whereas muscular or ligamentary stiffness is often felt as tension on the side opposite the movement.

Flexibility tests

A few tests to assess range of flexion at the hip, which can be taught in a class setting, are described below. These are informal, general tests, not precise diagnostic tools. If you notice any unusual restriction or pain in a student, especially in one hip compared to the other, don't hesitate to suggest consultation with a specialist.

The subject lies on his back, and uses the hands to flex the hip joint by pulling the knee toward the chest.

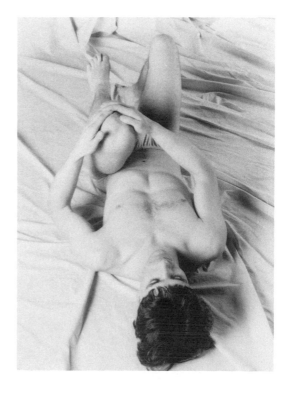

In "straight flexion" the anterior surfaces of the thigh and abdomen touch. The pelvis will be slightly tilted and the buttock slightly lifted off the floor.

In "crossed flexion" the knee is pulled toward the opposite shoulder. There is not as much contact between thigh and abdomen as in straight flexion.

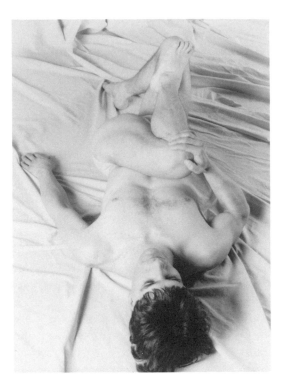

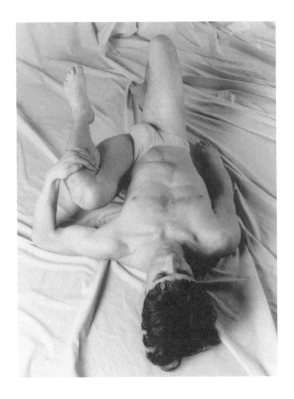

In "open flexion" the knee is pulled toward the ipsilateral shoulder. The thigh contacts the side of the body. In flexible individuals, the knee may be placed more or less in the armpit.

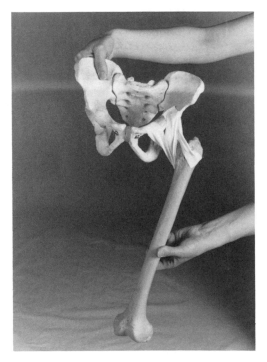

Ligamentary restrictions

Restrictions on movement at the hip arise mostly from associated ligaments and tendons, not the bones. Through knowledge of anatomy and common movements, we can predict which ligaments and muscles are more likely to stiffen.

The ligaments of the hip joint are more prominent anteriorly (see *AOM*, pp. 184–85). These thick ligaments are stretched by extension, retroversion, or lateral rotation, and tend to limit these movements. Extension and retroversion are a normal part of standing and walking.

In office workers, who spend long periods each day sitting, the hip stays flexed too long and the anterior ligaments tend to stiffen in a shortened position.

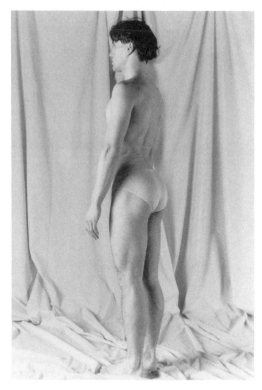

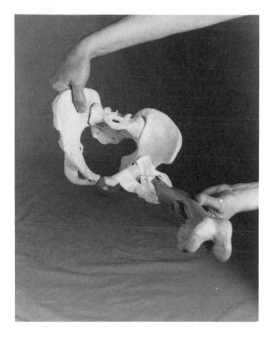

When the person tries to stand, extension at the hip is limited. To compensate, excessive lumbar arching may occur. This is unhealthy (see p. 34).

In contrast, consider the open flexion position (below, left). Here the anterior hip ligaments are continually stretched and do not stiffen. This is the position of the legs of babies carried on their mothers' backs, and also the position that most children adopt spontaneously when they play squatting down on the floor. If carried on into adulthood, this "frog" position greatly helps maintain flexibility of the anterior hip ligaments (below, right).

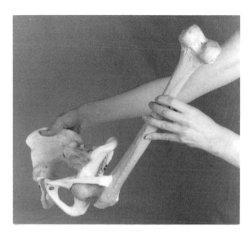

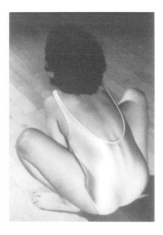

The exercises shown in our practice pages favor this position. Flexibility of the anterior ligaments also facilitates lateral rotation, which is important in ballet and martial arts.

Muscular restrictions

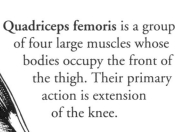

Quadriceps femoris is a group of four large muscles whose bodies occupy the front of the thigh. Their primary action is extension of the knee.

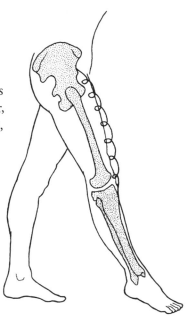

The three vastus muscles originate on the femur, but the fourth muscle, **rectus femoris**, originates on the ilium. It therefore crosses the hip joint as well as the knee joint (see *AOM*, p. 217) and can act as a hip flexor when the knee is fixed.

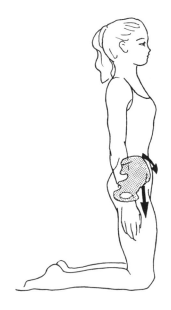

Tension on this muscle, as in hip extension, can take the pelvis into anteversion, particularly when the knee is flexed.

This tends to reinforce ligamentary stiffness as described above, and provoke compensatory (and undesirable) lumbar arching. It is important to keep the rectus femoris flexible through proper stretching exercises, some of which are presented in the practice pages.

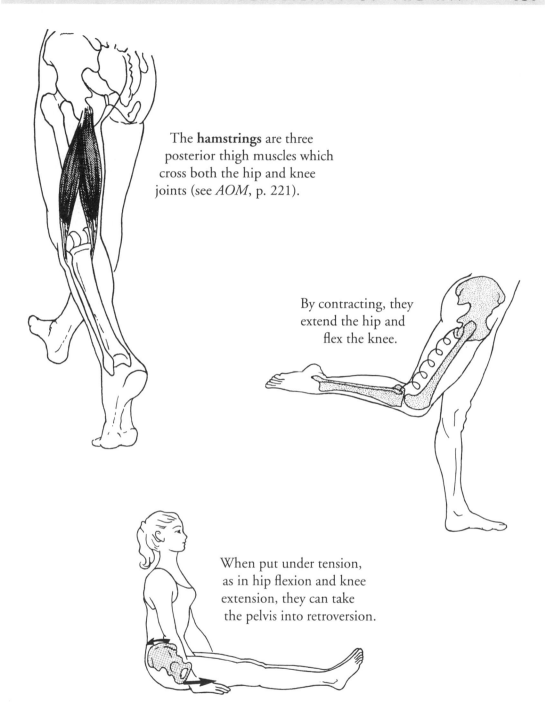

The **hamstrings** are three posterior thigh muscles which cross both the hip and knee joints (see *AOM*, p. 221).

By contracting, they extend the hip and flex the knee.

When put under tension, as in hip flexion and knee extension, they can take the pelvis into retroversion.

This may provoke rounding (flexion) of the lumbar spine, with consequent stress on the posterior spinal ligaments. "Tight" hamstrings are a common problem in modern society because people spend so much time sitting. This is frequently a contributing factor to lumbar back pain and bad posture. Exercises to keep the hamstrings supple and flexible are very important in physical movement classes. We believe even children should be taught how to stretch the hamstrings.

Tilting of the pelvis

Anteversion of the pelvis is encouraged by hip extension, because of tension on the iliofemoral ligament.

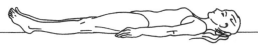

Examples are standing position,

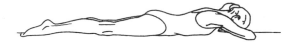

lying on the back or stomach with straight legs,

and kneeling with straight upper body.

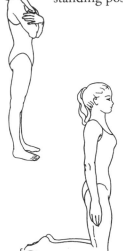

Pelvic anteversion is enhanced by knee flexion (because of stretching of the rectus femoris), as in lying prone with the hands grasping the feet.

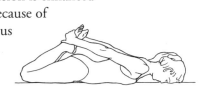

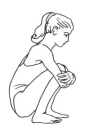

Retroversion of the pelvis is encouraged by hip flexion, especially past 90°, because of tension on the posterior ligaments and monoarticular muscles of the hip. Examples are squatting and sitting on the floor with knees bent.

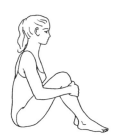

The retroversion may be enhanced by knee extension (because of tension on the hamstrings), as in lying down with legs against the wall, touching hands to the floor with straight legs, and sitting on the floor with legs straight.

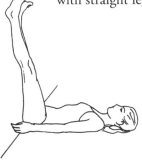

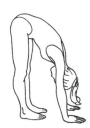

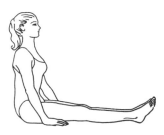

The pelvis is free to tilt forward or backward when the hip is in moderate flexion (which releases the rectus femoris) and the knee flexed (which releases the hamstrings),

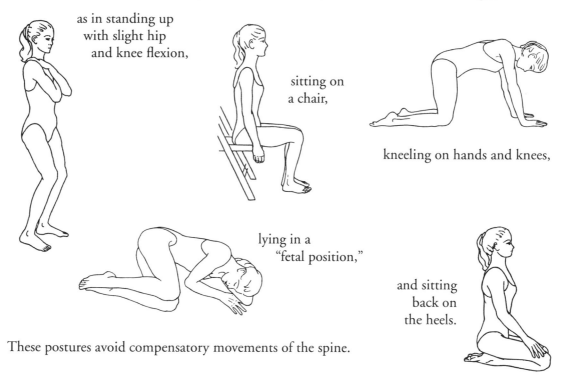

as in standing up with slight hip and knee flexion,

sitting on a chair,

kneeling on hands and knees,

lying in a "fetal position,"

and sitting back on the heels.

These postures avoid compensatory movements of the spine.

In certain asymmetrical movements and postures, the right and left halves of the pelvis behave differently. Examples are:

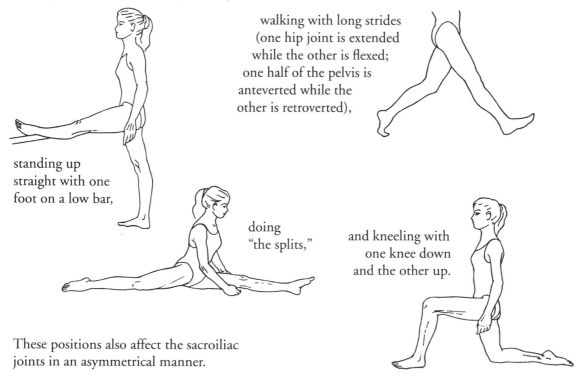

walking with long strides (one hip joint is extended while the other is flexed; one half of the pelvis is anteverted while the other is retroverted),

standing up straight with one foot on a low bar,

doing "the splits,"

and kneeling with one knee down and the other up.

These positions also affect the sacroiliac joints in an asymmetrical manner.

Muscular strength of the hip

Good ROM at the hip is desirable in terms of easy movement of the trunk and the legs. However, good strength and control of the muscles of the hip are also important. We face two general problems is designing and teaching exercise programs for this region:

- Most people do not have a clear mental picture of how the pelvis is shaped and oriented in three-dimensional space. They picture it as being more horizontal and flat than it really is. Both teachers and students are urged to palpate their own pelvic bones and look closely at a skeleton for better understanding.

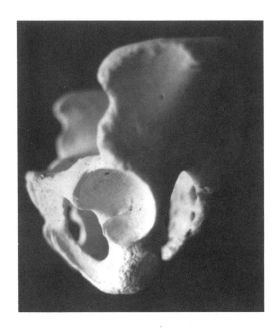

- The large muscle masses surrounding the hip joint make it impossible to palpate the joint or experience first-hand the way the femur articulates with the acetabulum. The shoulder, knee, and ankle joints are easier to palpate and understand.

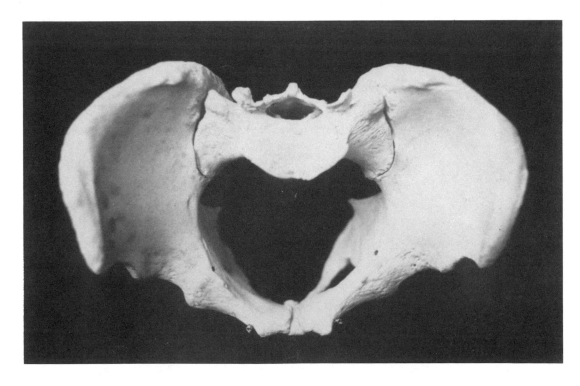

Deep muscles

It is useful for teaching purposes to distinguish the deep muscles of the hip from the superficial ones.

The deep muscles are relatively small and precise. They help fine-tune the orientation of the pelvis on the legs, and affect spinal curvatures. Their contraction tends to be chronic and prolonged. Important deep muscles are the obturator internus and externus, gemellus superior and inferior, quadratus femoris, gluteus minimus, and iliacus (see *AOM*, pp. 208–16). The first five are lateral rotators of the femur. When the femur is fixed, all seven can antevert or retrovert the pelvis. Their hammock- or basket-like arrangement (see pp. 176–79, and *AOM*, p. 212) helps to support and stabilize the pelvis.

Since these deep muscles are capable of "pulling apart" or decompressing the hip joint (see *AOM*, p. 212), appropriate exercises can relieve arthrosis caused by excessive compression.

Superficial muscles

These muscles are massive and powerful compared to the deep muscles. Their contraction tends to be intermittent rather than prolonged. We can view them as surrounding the hip and thigh on four sides:

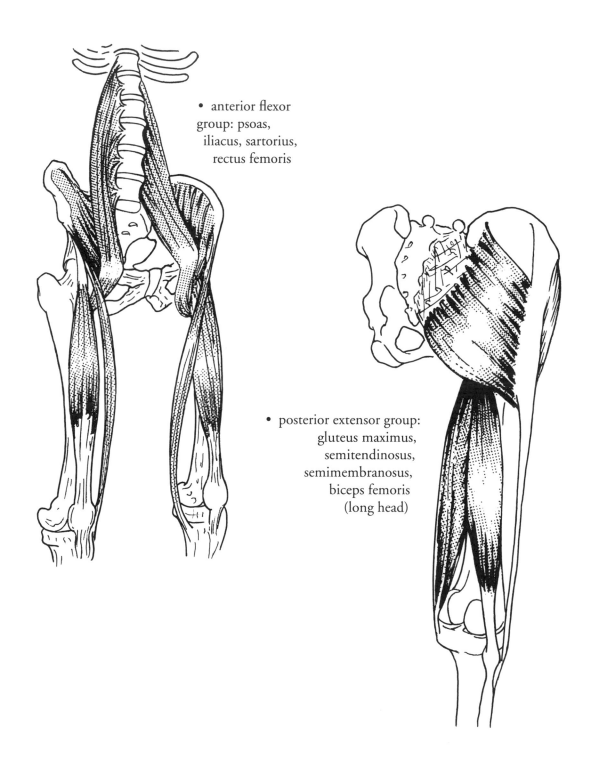

- anterior flexor group: psoas, iliacus, sartorius, rectus femoris

- posterior extensor group: gluteus maximus, semitendinosus, semimembranosus, biceps femoris (long head)

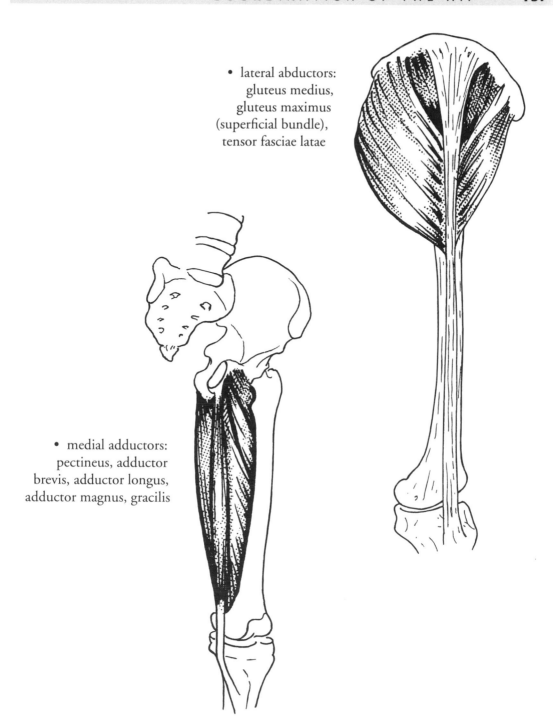

• lateral abductors:
gluteus medius,
gluteus maximus
(superficial bundle),
tensor fasciae latae

• medial adductors:
pectineus, adductor
brevis, adductor longus,
adductor magnus, gracilis

Coordination of the hip

The exercises in the following practice pages are concerned mainly with orientation of the pelvis on the femurs, and curvature of the spine in relation to the position of the pelvis. In the subsequent chapters on the knee and foot, we will focus more on coordination of hip muscles in movements of the leg.

Practice pages: Hip

Stretching the hip muscles

GENERAL STRETCHING*

The squatting position is adopted spontaneously by children all over the world when playing, and by adults in "primitive" cultures, but is generally avoided by teenagers and adults in Europe and North America. This is unfortunate, because it is a position which naturally increases flexibility. If you teach children, encourage them to adopt this position while listening or resting.

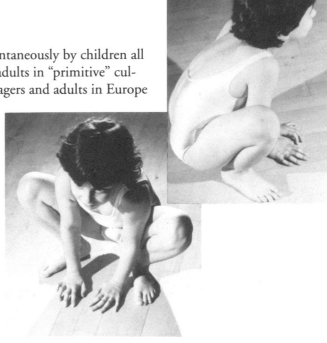

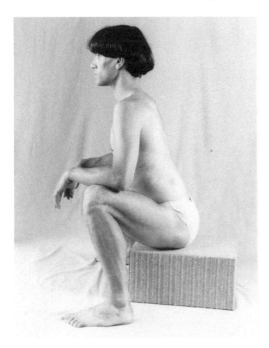

Adults will typically have lost some flexibility and therefore have difficulty maintaining this position. Two solutions are:

- Take the hip joint and muscles partly off-load by holding on to a bar or other support with the hands while squatting (do not encourage "bouncing," which serves no purpose).

- Sit on a low box or cushion (height of 8 inches or so).

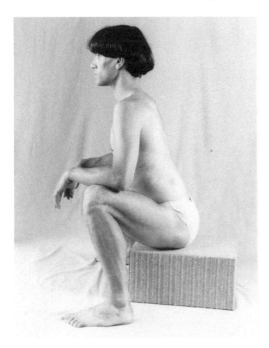
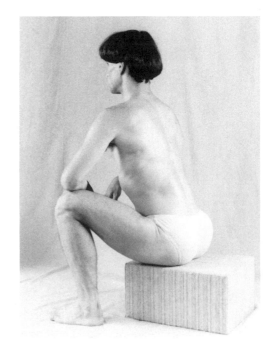

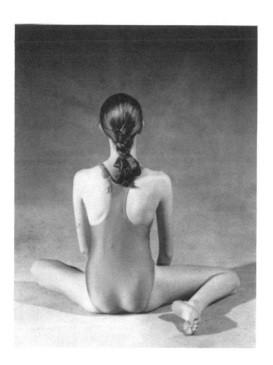

Put both legs flat on the floor, one in front of the pelvis and one behind, both bent at the knee. In these photos, the left and right hips are laterally and medially rotated respectively.

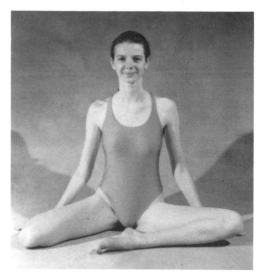

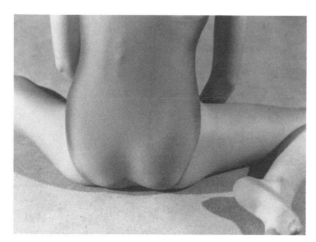

Both ischial tuberosities should be pressing down on something. For people who have lost hip flexibility, it will be very difficult to press the ischium of the "backward leg" against the floor.

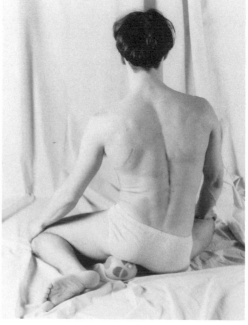

In this case, put some sort of cushion under that side, and progressively reduce the thickness of the support as flexibility improves. If there is difficulty getting one or both knees to touch the floor, press down on them with the hands.

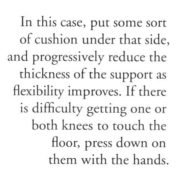

PASSIVE MOBILIZATION

Subject lies supine,
partner holds one leg
and moves the hip joint
in circumduction.

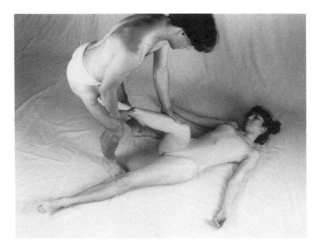

The knee should be
flexed to allow larger
ROM and less resistance.

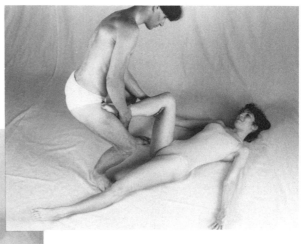

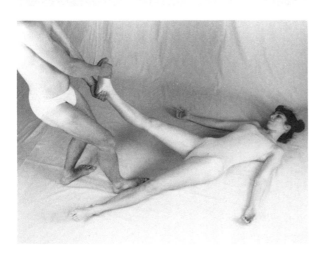

If the knee is extended,
ROM will typically be
limited by the hamstrings.

The partner can lightly
pull on the leg, either
while moving it as above,
or while it is stationary.

This mobilization should be done
slowly, in synchrony with breathing.
It is not a stretching exercise, and
no forceful pulling is needed.

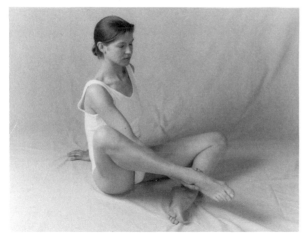

ACTIVE MOBILIZATION

Sit on the floor, left knee
flexed and off to the side.
Hold the right ankle or heel.

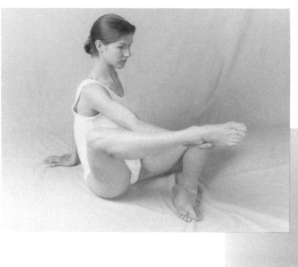

Move the right foot around such
that it "draws" an imaginary circle
in a sagittal plane, and then in a
frontal plane.

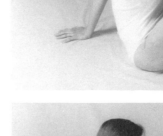

At first, keep ROM
small. If retroversion
of the pelvis occurs, use
the left hand for support.

Progressively work up to larger
ROM. Repeat the same process
with the left leg.

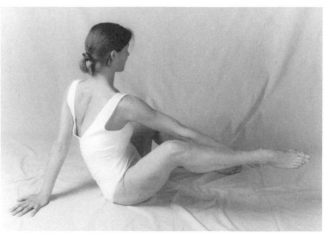

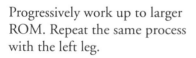

STRETCHING THE RECTUS FEMORIS*

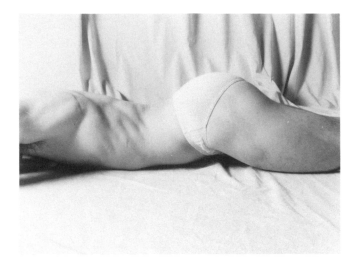

Lie on the stomach. Consciously antevert and retrovert the pelvis. In anteversion, the pubis moves away from the floor, while the anterior superior iliac spines (ASISs) move closer to the floor. In retroversion, the pubis moves closer and the ASISs move away from the floor.

Note that in retroversion the easiest contractions are those of the gluteals and rectus abdominis. Practice retroversion on one side only.

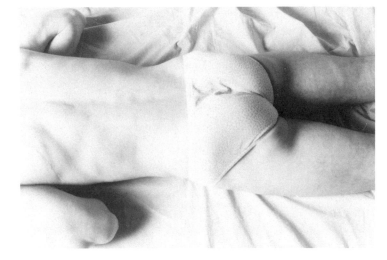

Flex the left knee and grasp the foot with the left hand.

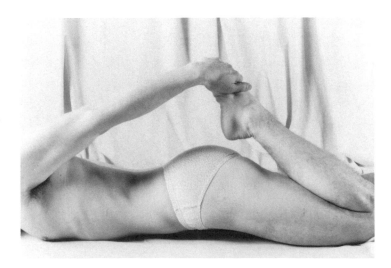

The rectus femoris is being stretched. Note that pelvic anteversion is occurring (the pubis is being lifted off the floor) on the left side.

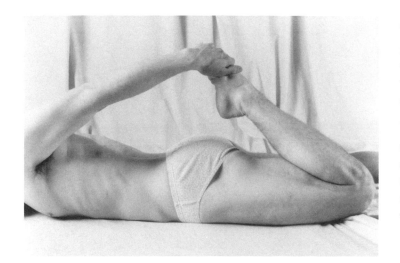

While still holding the foot, try to counteract the anteversion by contracting the rectus femoris or gluteus maximus.

You will feel a stretching sensation somewhere along the anterior thigh; the location of this sensation (inferior, middle, superior) varies from person to person.

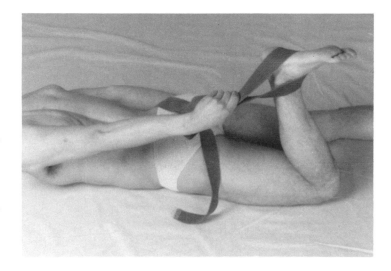

Extreme flexion of the knee (with pulling) can be harmful to people with a problem of the knee joint or kneecap. In these cases, the knee can be kept in moderate flexion by holding onto a strap,

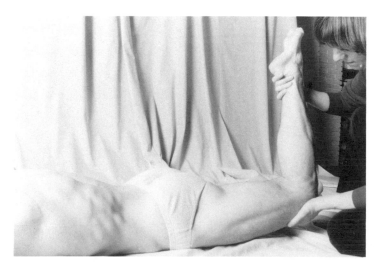

or having a partner hold the foot and knee.

STRETCHING THE HAMSTRINGS*

1. With the knee straight, put one foot on a stool or a bar.

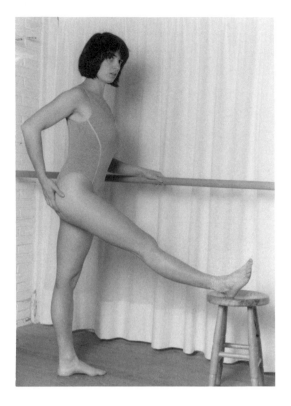

Make sure the pelvis stays anteverted, and the ischial tuberosities are directed posteroinferiorly. You can use a hand to maintain this orientation.

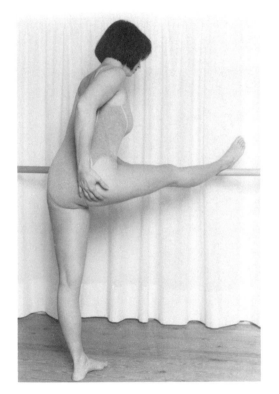

If you try to use a bar that is too high, the pelvis will inevitably go into retroversion, which defeats the purpose of this exercise.

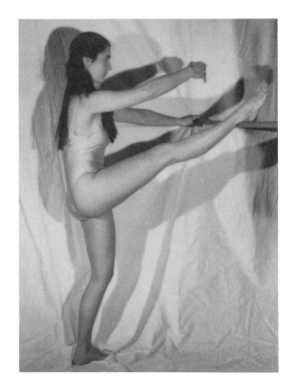

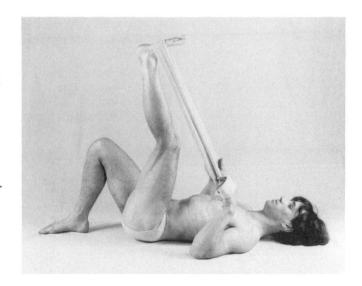

2. Lie on your back with
both hands holding
a strap which is passed
around the foot. Hold
the foot so it is directly
above the hip joint
(if necessary, bend
the knee slightly).

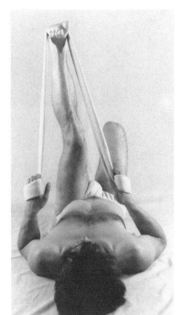

Try to simultaneously press the coccyx against the floor
and dorsiflex the ankle (which will tend to extend the knee).
Eliminate compensatory movements such as medial rotation
of the femur (you will see the kneecap directed medially),

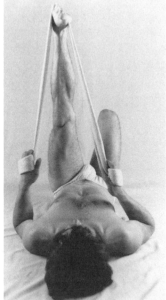

or inversion
of the foot.

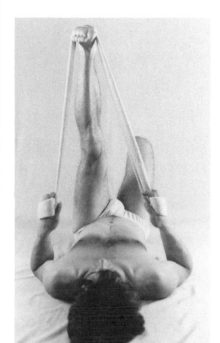

The correct position
is with both the knee
and foot straight.

3. Sit with feet against the wall and knees straight.

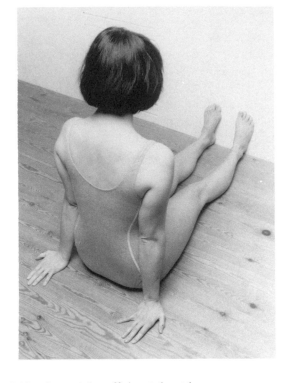

Take the weight off the right side by leaning on the left hand. Use the right hand to pull the right ischial tuberosity farther away from the wall while keeping the right foot in place.

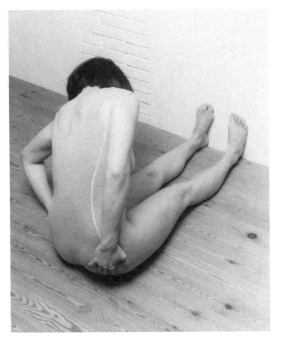

Put the weight back on the right side. Repeat this process for the left ischial tuberosity. The overall result here is stretching of the hamstrings.

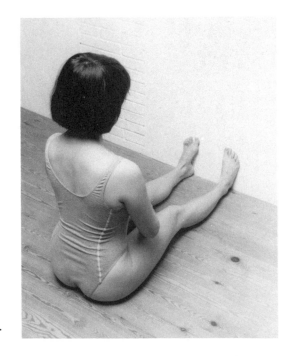

Ideally, we want to minimize the small concavity (lumbar lordosis) just above the sacrum.

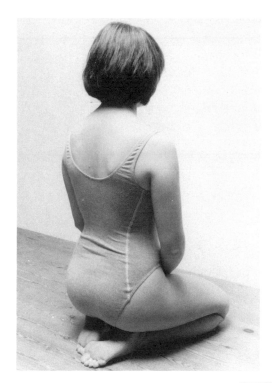

It may be helpful, before performing this exercise, to familiarize yourself with the location of this concavity by assuming a position where it is prominent (e.g., sitting on the heels), and feeling it with the hands.

For beginners, the correct positioning of the legs and pelvis is most important. Reduction of the lumbar concavity is of secondary importance.

As in the preceding exercise, it is essential to avoid compensating movements such as medial rotation of the femurs or inversion of the feet.

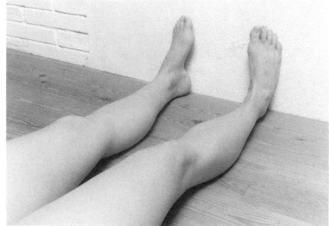

In the correct position, the kneecaps point straight up and both feet are flat against the wall.

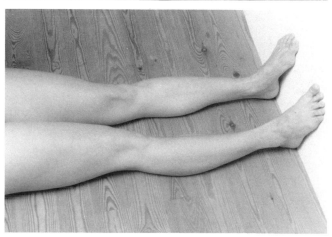

STRETCHING THE ADDUCTORS AND ROTATORS

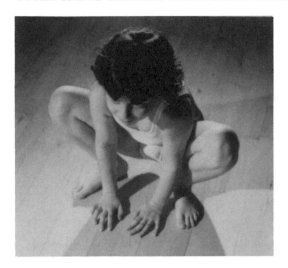

Most of these muscles are stretched in the squatting position. However, because of the flexion of the knee, the gracilis (an adductor) is not stretched.

To stretch the gracilis, extend the knees and spread the legs wide apart. Try to sit on the ischial tuberosities. If this is difficult, leave the pelvis in retroversion, and put more of your weight on the hands.

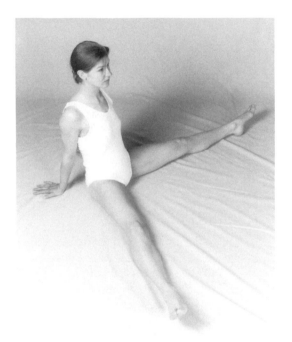

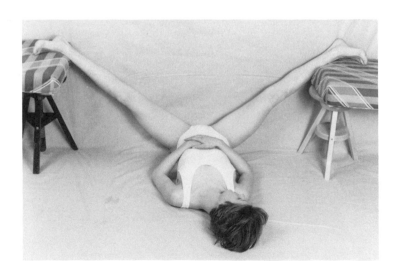

A variation on the above exercise requires two props. Lie on your back with knees extended, legs spread, and the feet resting against the wall and against two supports as shown. Position the supports for maximal stretching of the muscles.

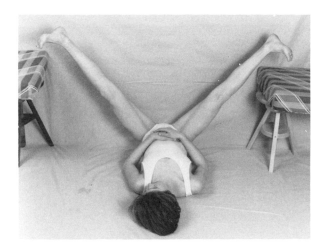

You may find that the two legs do not spread to the same degree. You can allow this asymmetry while still keeping the pelvis pressed symmetrically against the floor by carefully modifying the position of the two supports. First, lift the feet off the supports, move the supports closer together, and contract the adductors and rotators by doing medial or lateral hip rotations. Next, relax the adductors and put the feet back on the supports. Tilt the pelvis in all possible directions:

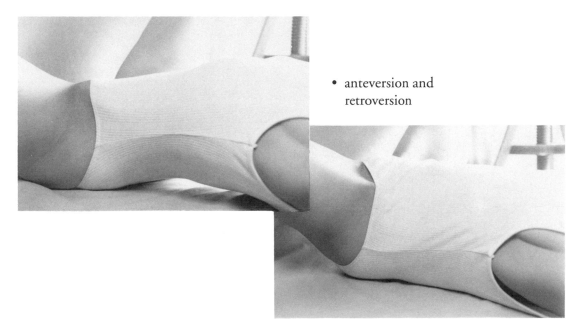

- anteversion and retroversion

- abduction/adduction (see pp. 142–43)

- medial/lateral rotation (see p. 144).

These movements stretch all the layers and groups of adductor and rotator muscles. Progressively move the two supports apart from each other until the optimal position for each leg is achieved.

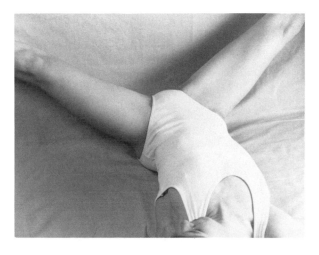

STRETCHING THE ABDUCTORS

Lie on your back and cross one leg over the other. Exert pressure of the two ankles against each other. At the same time, move the pelvis in anteversion/retroversion and medial/lateral rotation, as in the preceding exercise.

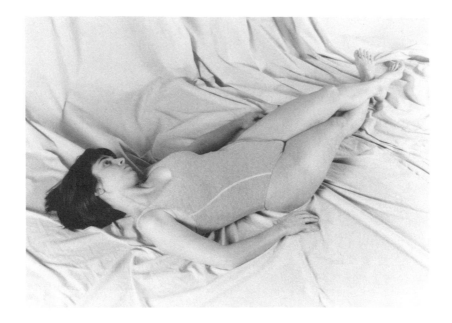

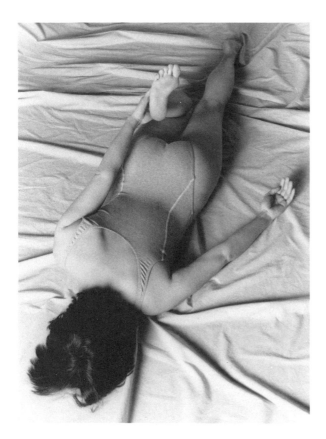

To stretch the tensor fasciae latae, lie on your stomach and repeat the exercise described for the rectus femoris (see p. 162), with strong adduction of the flexed knee against the extended leg.

Strengthening the hip muscles

STRENGTHENING THE DEEP MUSCLES

Lie on your back and raise both flexed knees above the abdomen. Place your hands on the outsides of the knees as shown, then try to abduct the knees against the resistance with the hands.

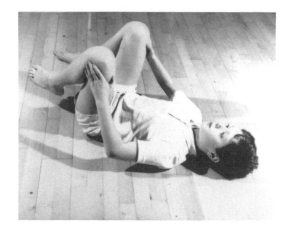

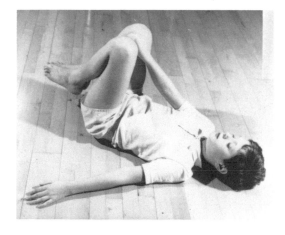

The six deep muscles shown on p. 155, which are mainly rotators of the hip, are being activated here. However, the gluteal muscles are also involved, and we want to relax them in order to isolate the six rotators.

Place one fist between the knees and adduct the knees strongly against it.

Next, place the hands flat just proximal to the knees. Flex the thighs against the resistance of the hands. The iliacus and psoas are working here. To work the psoas more specifically, concentrate on pressing the lumbar spine against the floor.

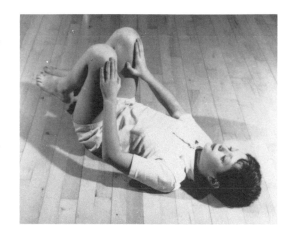

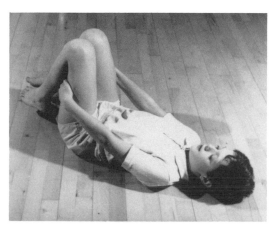

Finally, wrap the hands around the posterior thighs. Extend the thighs against the resistance of the hands. Try to relax the gluteal muscles as much as possible so that the deep muscles are doing most of the work.

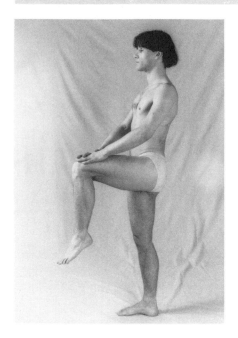

STRENGTHENING THE FLEXORS

Stand on one leg. You can lean against a wall or bar to keep your balance. Flex the other hip and knee and press up against the resistance of the hands.

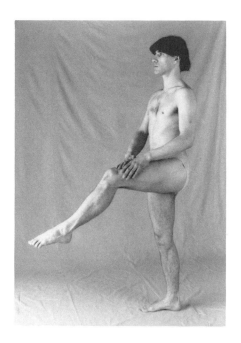

You can increase the difficulty by trying to extend the knee. This gets the hamstrings involved.

Next, move the hand somewhat laterally on the knee and press in that direction, which recruits the abductors.

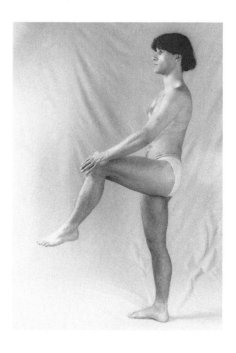

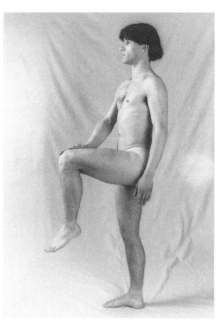

Next, move the hand on the medial side of the knee and press in that direction to recruit the adductors.

You can get the psoas involved by trying to straighten out the lumbar curve at the same time you flex the hip.

STRENGTHENING THE EXTENSORS

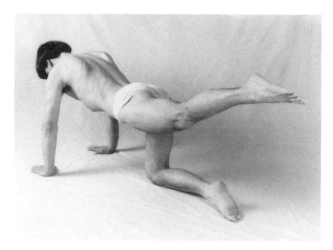

Start in the hand-knee position, back straight, and raise one leg as high as possible, foot plantar flexed.

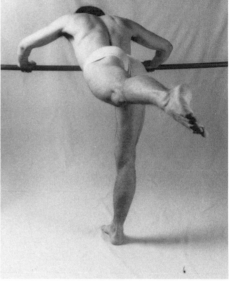

In an alternative exercise, stand on one leg, hold onto a bar, and raise the other leg.

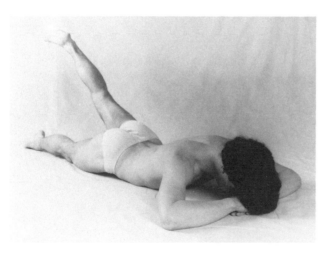

Lie prone, raise each leg in turn and hold it up, keeping the pelvis in retroversion the whole time.

In these exercises, the femur can be in neutral or lateral rotation. In the latter case, the gluteus maximus works harder. Try to keep the pelvis in a fixed position, although this is very difficult.

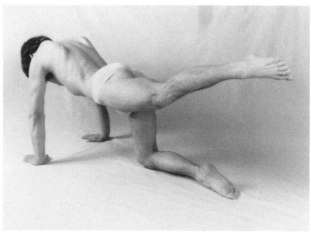

STRENGTHENING THE ABDUCTORS AND ROTATORS

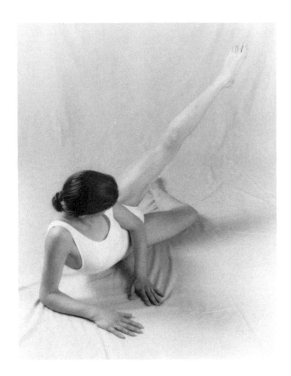

Lie on one side, using the extended or flexed bottom leg for support. You can lean on one elbow or press the whole side against the floor. Raise the upper leg off the floor in neutral rotation, knee straight, and flex the hip slightly. Rotate the femur medially (works the gluteus minimus and anterior bundle of gluteus medius) and then laterally (tensor fasciae latae).

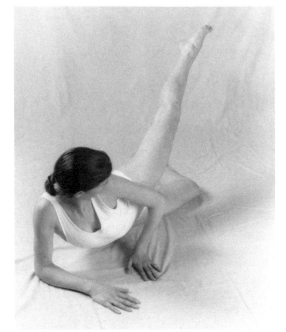

Extend the hip slightly and rotate the femur some more (involves gluteus maximus).

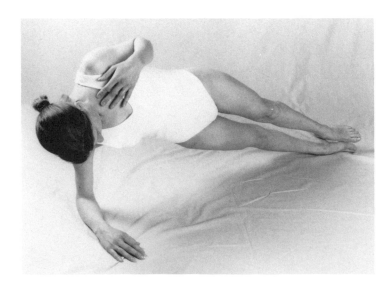

To increase difficulty, repeat these exercises with pelvis and torso lifted off the floor, and all your weight supported by one forearm and foot.

STRENGTHENING THE ADDUCTORS AND ROTATORS

Lie on your back, hips flexed, knees straight, feet dorsiflexed and pointing straight up. Have the feet separated by a folded cloth or a partner's hands.

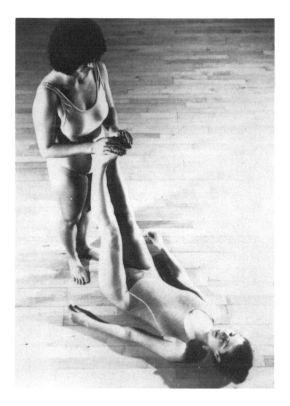

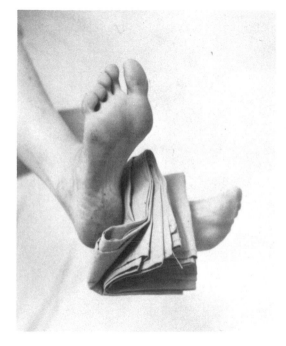

Work the adductors and gracilis by pressing the knees and feet together. Next, focus on pressing the heels together (posterior adductors).

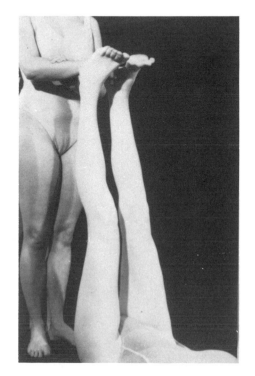

Finally, press the big toes together (anterior adductors).

Coordination of hip muscles

ANTEVERSION/ RETROVERSION

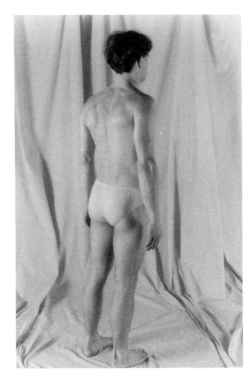

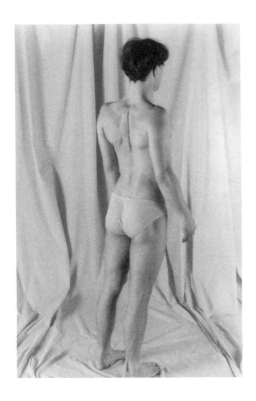

Stand with hips, knees, and ankles slightly flexed. This position facilitates free movement of the pelvis (see p. 153). Practice anteverting and retroverting the pelvis.

Note that anteversion can be associated with arching (lordosis) of the lumbar spine, and retroversion with flattening of the lumbar curve.

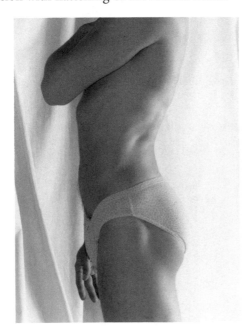

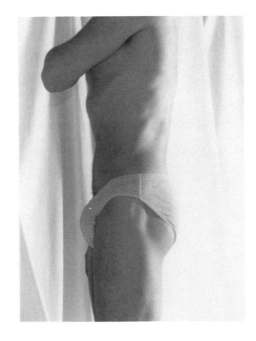

At the same time, realize that these lumbar spine movements are distinct from the pelvic movements and involve different muscles.

Feel the large muscles involved in anteversion:
- rectus femoris (sensation of contraction at anterior thigh)
- iliacus (sensation inside iliac "wings")
- lumbar spinal muscles.

The large superficial muscles involved in retroversion are the gluteals and rectus abdominis.

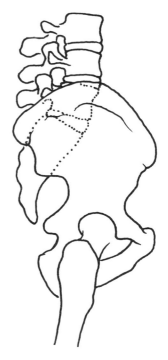

Next, try to relax all the muscles just mentioned, yet continue tilting the pelvis back and forth, under control of the deep muscles: piriformis (see *AOM*, p. 209), quadratus femoris, obturator internus and externus, gemellus superior and inferior (see p. 155). These muscles have small ROM and will give sensations of minimal contraction, located deeply. Piriformis moves the sacrum in a plane parallel to the femur.

Impose two limits for the pelvic tilting:

For anteversion, stop before you feel posterior pressure at the L5-S1 joint.

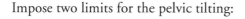

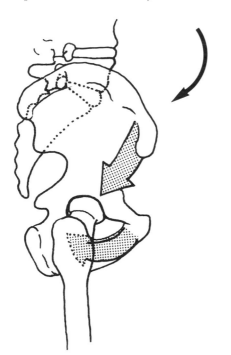

For retroversion, stop when you feel that the lumbar curve has been straightened.

The deep muscles are constantly adjusting the position of the pelvis during walking, standing, kneeling, etc. By being aware of these subtle movements and exercising the muscles, you promote the proper posture, functioning, and health of the hip joints and spine.

HORIZONTAL MOVEMENTS OF THE PELVIS

The pelvis can move in a horizontal plane, like a drawer being pulled in and out:

• anteriorly   • posteriorly

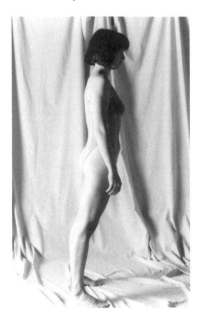 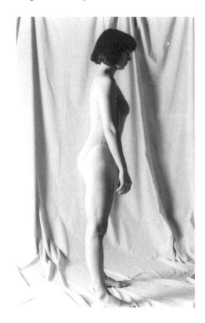

This type of movement should affect the legs but not the orientation of the spine. Make sure to localize it at the level of the femoral heads, *not* in the lumbar region, where the tendency would be to:

• arch the lumbar spine   • contract the gluteals
  (lordosis)   (flattening the lumbar curve)

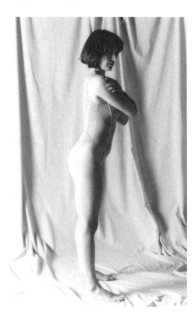 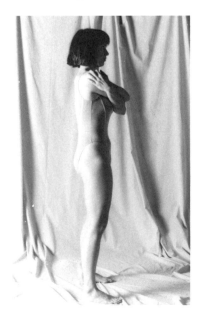

Start out working with the strongest muscles, then try to progressively relax them and work at a deeper level, with decreased ROM and more subtle movements. The pelvis uses these horizontal movements to find its "balance" on the femurs, like a person walking on stilts. This happens especially in babies just before they learn to walk, when they practice extending the knees and hips and putting more body weight on the feet.

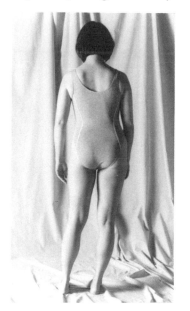

You can also shift the pelvis laterally in a horizontal plane.

In a related exercise, you lift one foot and swing the pelvis on the supporting leg:

• forward

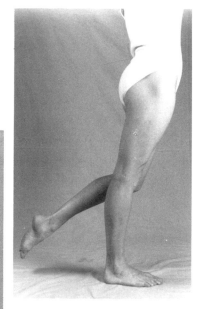

• to the left

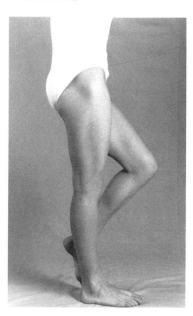

• backward

• to the right

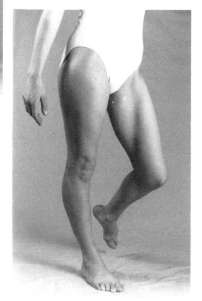

The pelvis is essentially circumducting on the supporting leg. This is a good exercise for improving balance.

CHAPTER SEVEN

The Knee

....

The knee, like its counterpart the elbow, is basically a hinge joint allowing a large range of flexion. The degree of flexion is small during walking, and larger in activities such as running, kneeling, sitting, and jumping. In contrast to the elbow, flexion of the knee is sometimes associated with slight rotation (see *AOM*, pp. 197–202). Muscular strength is essential for stability of the knee.

Movements

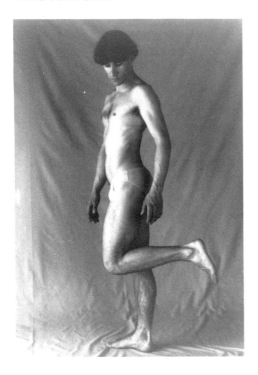

In **flexion** the posterior surfaces of the thigh and leg move closer together.

Typical examples are the plié in ballet, landing after a jump, and walking up stairs.

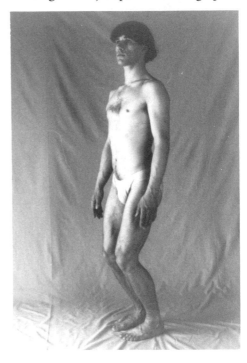

At the extreme range of flexion, the muscular masses of the posterior thigh and calf are compressed against each other.

Typically, the femur and tibia move simultaneously in flexion, e.g., in a plié. The femur can remain fixed while the tibia moves, as in a backward kicking movement. Knee flexion with the tibia fixed and the femur moving is theoretically possible but rarely happens in real life. One example would be having your legs buried in sand at the beach and then lowering yourself to a sitting position.

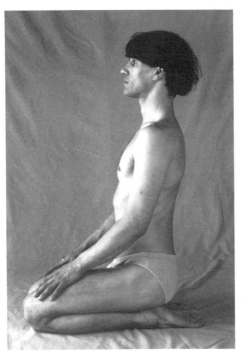

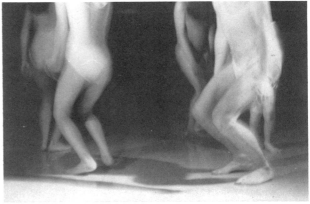

In **extension** the knee joint returns from a
flexed position to a straight (anatomical)
position. This movement can be observed
during walking, standing on tiptoe,
coming up from a plié, kicking a ball.

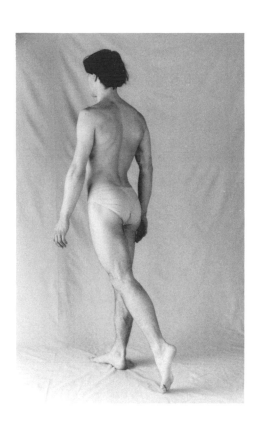

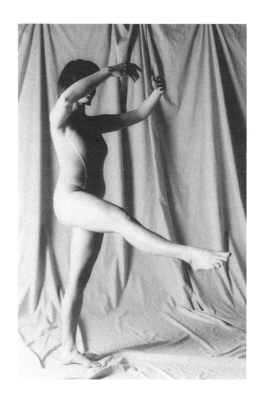

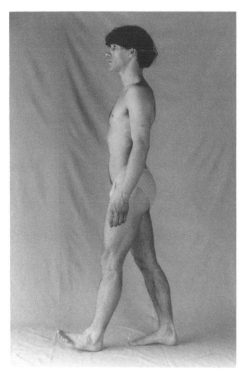

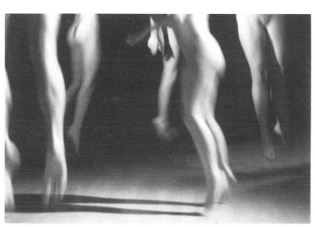

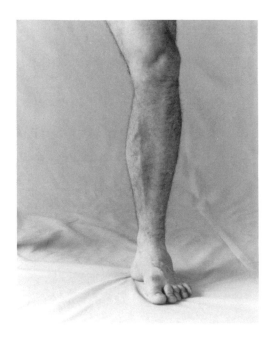

Slight **rotation** is possible when the knee is flexed, since this causes slackening of the ligaments which otherwise prevent rotation.

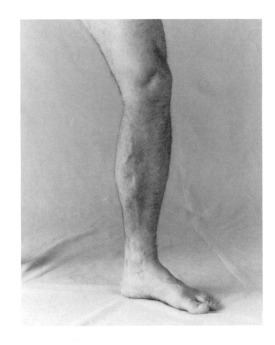

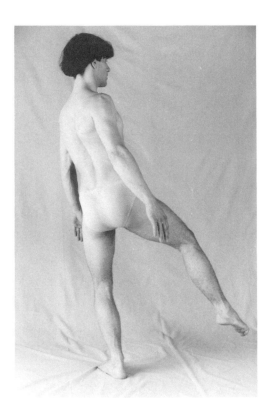

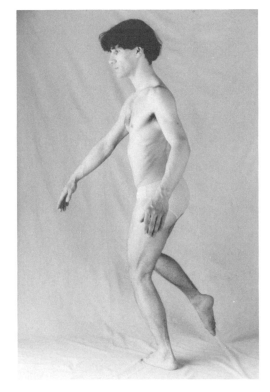

Be careful not to confuse knee rotation with hip or ankle rotation (see *AOM*, p. 207). If you plant one foot on the ground, flex the ipsilateral knee, and lift the other foot off the ground, you will see that some rotation is possible.

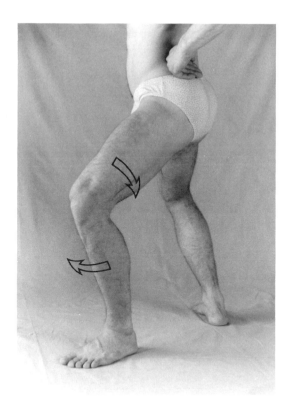

"Automatic" rotation of the knee occurs in combination with flexion and extension, because of the shape of the femoral and tibial condyles and the relative strength of the medial and lateral collateral ligaments (see *AOM*, p. 202). During a plié, for instance, the knee is flexing and the femur and tibia undergo slight lateral and medial rotation respectively.

As the knee is straightened, the reverse occurs. These knee rotations, although they have a very small ROM, are essential to proper movement of the hip joint and placement of the foot in walking.

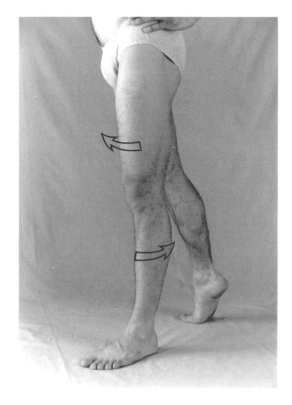

Bones of the knee

Alignment of the femur and tibia

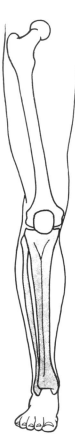

These two long bones form a column supporting the weight of the upper body. Their alignment is not perfectly straight. The "mechanical axis" passing through the femoral head and the ankle joint is about 3° off from a sagittal plane, and the axes defined by the shafts of the two long bones typically form a lateral angle of 170°–175° rather than 180° (see *AOM*, p. 194). Cases in which this angle is significantly below or above this range are termed "genu valgum" and "genu varum" respectively.

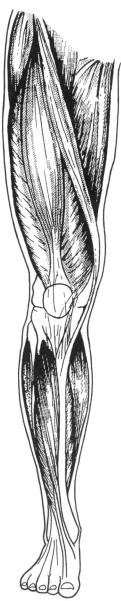

These bone alignments are easily seen in X-rays, but are obscured to the naked eye by the position of the large muscle masses. The femur is located laterally in relation to the large masses of the quadriceps and hamstrings, whereas the tibia is medial relative to the large calf muscles.

Bone growth

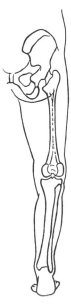

The femur and tibia increase tremendously in length between infancy and adulthood. Most of this growth occurs in parts of the bones near the knee joint. As with all long bones, longitudinal growth of the femur and tibia takes place at the epiphysial cartilages, located at the junctions of the epiphyses (expanded ends of the bone) and the diaphysis (central shaft).

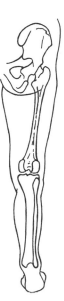

Bone growth is most rapid from birth until age five. During this period, genu valgum and genu varum are common and typically reversible.

Growth continues, but usually at slower rates, until age 17 or so. Correct alignment of the leg bones and distribution of stresses on the tibial plateau promote the harmonious growth of the epiphysial cartilages. If you conduct exercise classes for children below age 10, you should explain the correct alignment of the bones and train the children to feel and see important bony landmarks. We recommend three types of exercises:

- non-weight bearing exercises for alignment of the knees, malleoli, and feet (see pp. 242–45).
- standing on one leg or both legs, with awareness of bone alignment and position of the bony landmarks; don't stay in a static position for too long, however
- coordination of basic movements of the hip, knee, and foot (see p. 247).

Flexibility of the knee

Ligamentary flexibility

In contrast to the elbow, the knee does not rely on bone shapes to restrict movement. The patella does not act as a "brake" to knee extension. It is not closely fitted to the femur and tibia. Restrictions to movement, and stability of the joint, result mainly from the arrangement of ligaments around the knee. When we speak of flexibility here, we don't mean that we want to elongate the ligaments. Rather, we want to preserve normal ROM.

In full flexion, the anterior knee capsule and ligaments are completely "unfolded" whereas the posterior capsule is folded on itself.

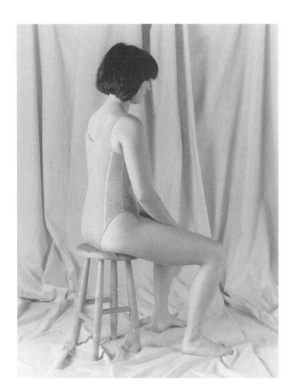

Flexion ROM may be reduced by some trauma to the capsule, yet still be sufficient for common daily activities, at least in Western countries where 90° flexion is enough.

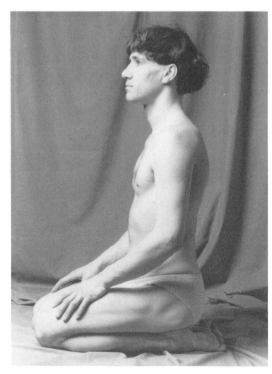

In Eastern countries (where squatting or sitting on the heels is common), or in physical disciplines, full flexion is required.

In extension, the femur and tibia go back to forming a straight line, at least when seen from the side. The brake to hyperextension comes from the posterior knee capsule, which is very thick. We sometimes see a looseness of the posterior capsule, particularly in children, which allows some hyperextension of the knee ("recurvatum").

The knee should never sidebend. If it does, this is a pathological condition resulting from looseness or overstretching of the collateral ligaments and causing serious instability of the knee. Avoid any exercise which stretches the collateral ligaments! When the tibia laterally rotates under the femur, or the femur medially rotates on the tibia, the collateral ligaments are pulled straight (see *AOM*, p. 200). You should therefore avoid forcing this type of rotation (torques), especially in weight-bearing situations.

Sitting on the floor with the flexed legs to either side requires good medial rotation of the hip. Children are able to do this easily because their hip joints are very flexible.

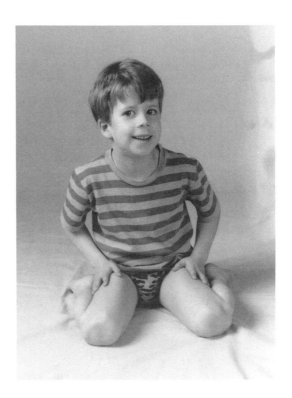

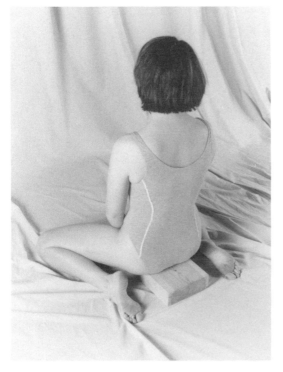

In adults with reduced flexibility, medial rotation of the hip is insufficient, and attempts to sit this way force lateral rotation (and pain) of the tibia at the knee. If this happens, change position immediately and work on increasing flexibility of the hip. A support under the ischial tuberosities can also take the stress off the knees.

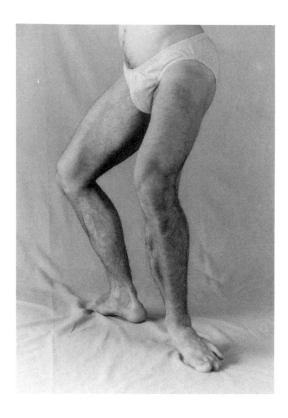

A similarly harmful exercise
is forced lateral rotation of
the foot when lateral rotation
at the hips is insufficient.
In the plié shown, the knee
is above the medial foot.

The tibia is being laterally
rotated on the femur, and the
medial collateral ligament is
being harmfully stretched,
especially if we jump or
spin in this position,
or stand on one foot.

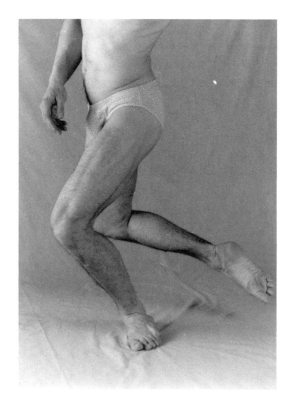

Muscular flexibility

The knee is spanned by the rectus femoris anteriorly and the hamstrings posteriorly. Stretching these muscles is important for maintaining good flexibility. The hamstrings can exert a strong braking action on complete extension of the knee. Three conditions may be encountered:

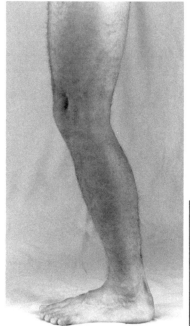

- "Flexum." It is difficult to completely straighten the knee, even passively. Fairly common in older adults, very rare in children. Treatment requires stretching the posterior knee (hamstrings) with monoarticular movements, or polyarticular movements involving the hip and ankle.

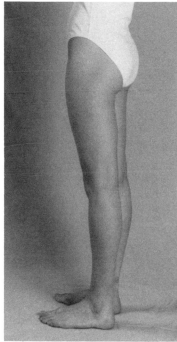

- Knee extends to a normal 180° angle. Most frequent condition. Should be maintained.

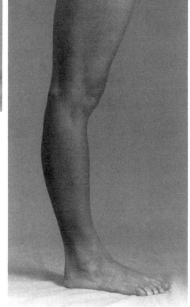

- Hyperextension (recurvatum) of the knee. Results from looseness of the posterior ligaments and capsule. Passive hyperextension of the knee in these cases stretches the cruciate ligaments and should be avoided.

Muscular strength of the knee

As explained above, stability of the knee is based not on bone shapes but on the ligamentary (passive) and muscular (active) attachments of the joint. In strengthening the muscles around the knee, we improve the stability of the joint as well as facilitate specific movements required by physical disciplines.

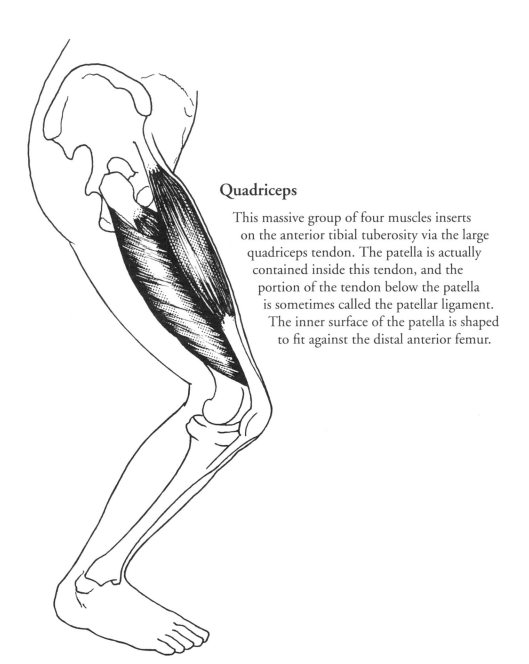

Quadriceps

This massive group of four muscles inserts on the anterior tibial tuberosity via the large quadriceps tendon. The patella is actually contained inside this tendon, and the portion of the tendon below the patella is sometimes called the patellar ligament. The inner surface of the patella is shaped to fit against the distal anterior femur.

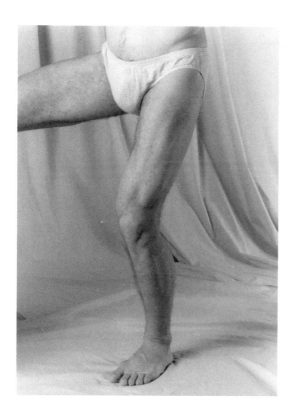

The quadriceps, the strongest muscles in the body, are extensors of the leg. They are involved in kicking movements, holding the extended leg, coming up from a plié, providing the propulsive force for jumping, etc.

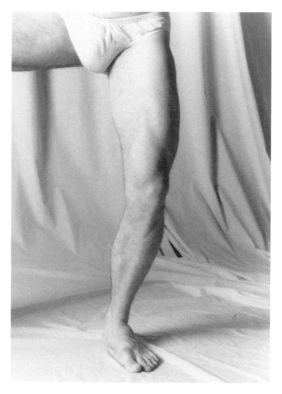

Proper relation of the patella to the femur is important for functioning of the quadriceps (see *AOM*, pp. 203–04). In adults, femoral-patellar arthrosis (particularly on the lateral side) frequently causes pain.

We can deal with this by strengthening the muscles to take stress off the femoral-patellar cartilages, and by developing better coordination between muscles of the hip, knee, and foot.

Medial and posteromedial muscles

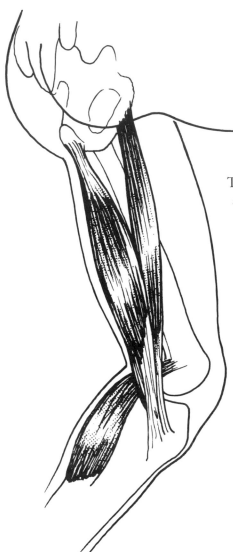

This group includes gracilis, semitendinosus, semimembranosus, and the medial origin of gastrocnemius. These muscles serve as "active ligaments" of the knee, reinforcing the medial collateral ligament. In this role, they are more important than their lateral counterparts.

The fact that the femur and tibia form a lateral angle of 170°–175° rather than 180° (see p. 186) means that the knee joint tends to be compressed on the lateral side and "open" on the medial side, requiring stronger medial support.

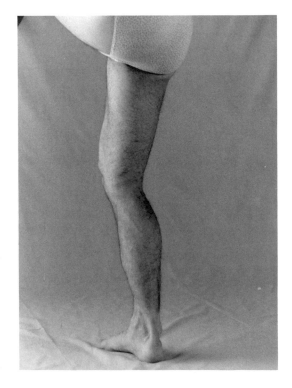

Lateral and posterolateral muscles

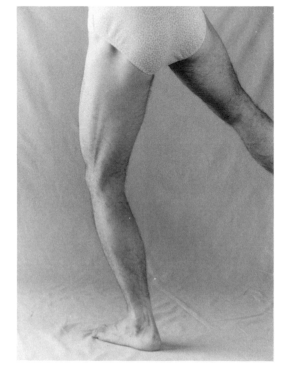

This group consists of tensor fasciae latae, biceps femoris, and the lateral origin of gastrocnemius. They reinforce the lateral collateral ligament and promote lateral stability of the knee and the entire leg during walking.

These muscles are like reins guiding the tibia in rotation from the back, and also play a role in positioning of the ankle (see p. 219).

Practice pages: Knee

Flexibility

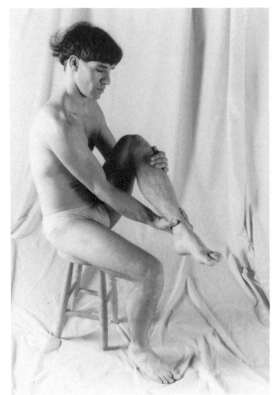

FLEXION-EXTENSION

A person who cannot flex the knee completely generally needs to be referred to a physical therapist. However, if there is no pain, try this simple exercise. Sit down, flex the knee, and hold the ankle with one hand. Gradually increase flexion while making slow, slight rotations of the tibia. This distributes synovial fluid through the joint cavity and moves the menisci in a beneficial way.

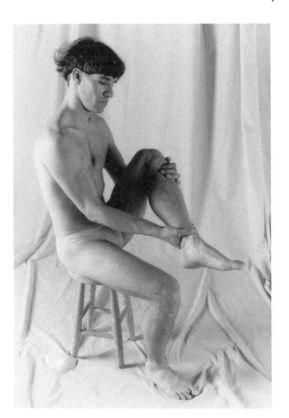

PASSIVE MOVEMENT
OF THE PATELLA

The patella cannot be moved when the knee is flexed (because it is then held between the femoral condyles) or when the quadriceps is activated (because of tension of the quadriceps tendon). Movement of the patella requires that the knee be in passive extension. Sit on the floor with legs stretched out straight.

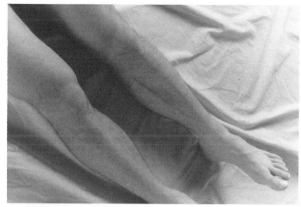

You will be able to move the patellas around easily with the hands:

• from side to side

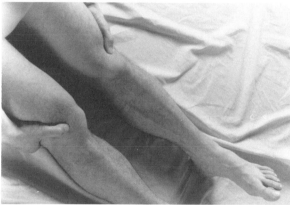

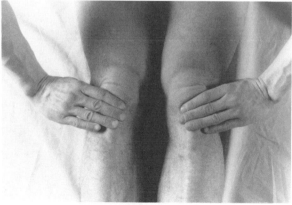

• superiorly

• inferiorly

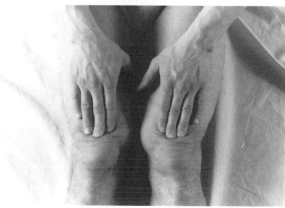

This causes slight articular decompression and good movement of the synovial fluid. Avoid pressing the patella against the femur!

Muscular stretching

Many of the exercises described for the
hip joint apply to the knee as well, e.g.,
stretching of the:

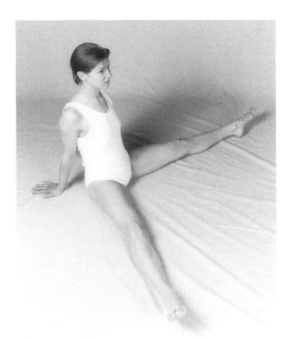

- adductors
  (see p. 168)

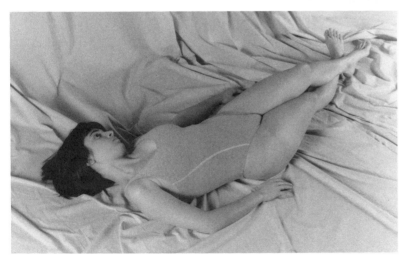

- abductors
  (see p. 170)

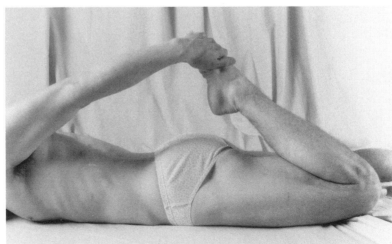

- rectus femoris
  (see p. 162)

- hamstrings (see pp. 164–67).

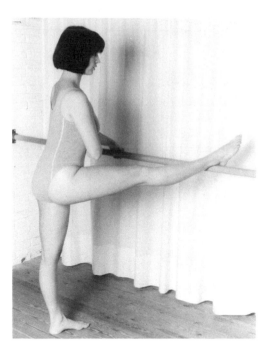

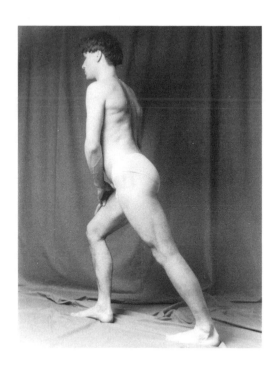

Stretching exercises for the ankle are also helpful for the knee (see p. 224–25).

The hamstrings and gastrocnemius can be stretched simultaneously by a combination of hip flexion, knee extension, and ankle dorsiflexion. For example:

- Sit on the floor and strongly flex the feet and toes.

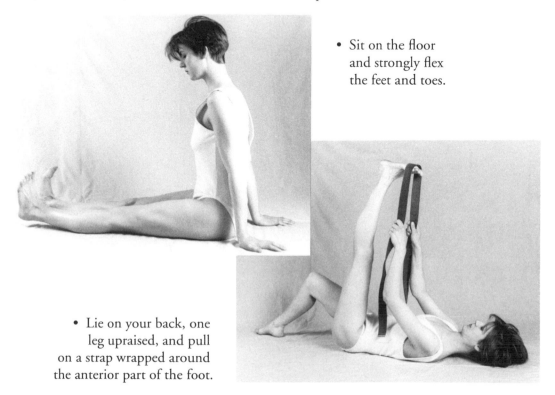

- Lie on your back, one leg upraised, and pull on a strap wrapped around the anterior part of the foot.

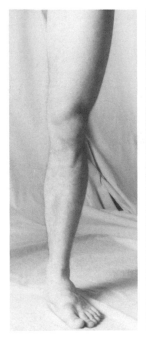
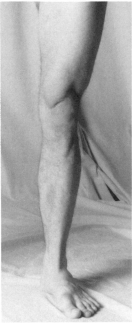

Muscular strengthening

QUADRICEPS

These muscles are easy
to visualize because
when they contract,
the patella moves up.

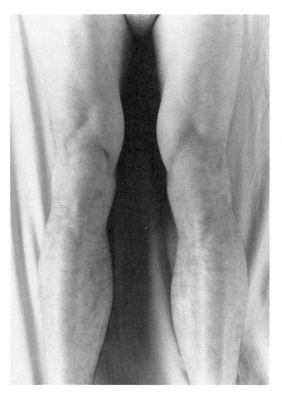

With your eyes closed,
move the patella up and
down in order to imprint
this sensation in your body.
It may be easier to do this
sitting down with legs
stretched out. This feeling
and its visualization help
you to be "in control," and
know whether the knee is
in full or partial extension.

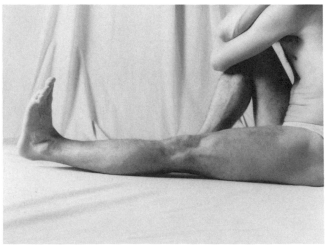

Sit down with one knee
upraised and the other
extended. Contract the
quadriceps such that the
back of the knee moves
closer to the floor and
the heel rises off the floor.

Try to differentiate the contraction of the four heads. The contraction of the vastus intermedius muscle is medial and deep, and can be felt even at the back of the femur.

To appreciate the contraction of the vastus muscles, have a partner push against one side or the other of your foot, and resist this rotation.

When the lateral side of the foot is pressed, the vastus lateralis contracts to resist the medial rotation of the hip.

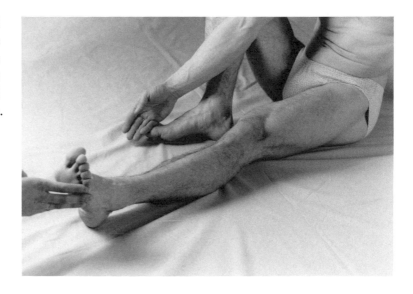

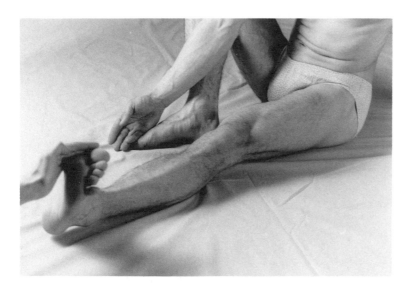

When the medial side of the foot is pressed, the vastus medialis contracts to resist the lateral rotation of the hip.

Strengthening of vastus medialis is helpful in relieving arthrosis of the femoral-patellar area (see *AOM*, pp. 203–04).

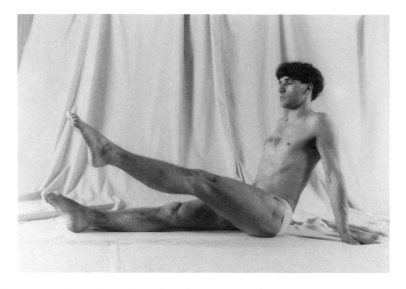

Finally, lift the entire leg off the floor (hip flexion) with knee extended. Here the rectus femoris is working in addition to the three vastus. Resistance is provided by the hamstrings, which are being stretched by the hip flexion and try to flex the knee.

For a static quadriceps exercise, lean against a wall or partner's back with hips and knees flexed. Experiment to find the position where the muscles are working hardest. To increase the difficulty, lift one foot off the floor.

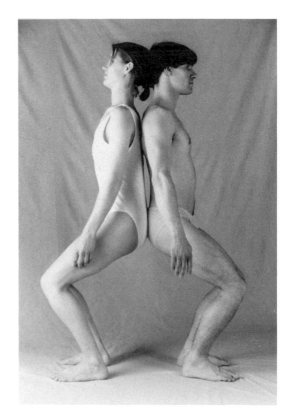

OTHER MUSCLES

Again, certain hip exercises are applicable to the knee as well:

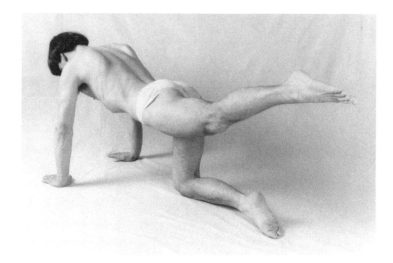

- posterior muscles
  (extensors)
  (see p. 173)

- lateral muscles
  (abductors)
  (see p. 174)

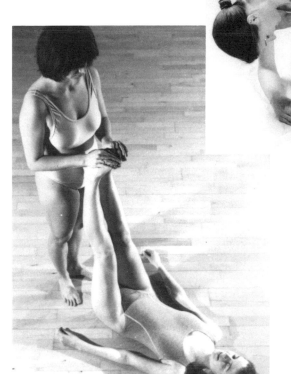

- medial muscles
  (adductors)
  (see p. 175)

Muscular coordination

When the knee is flexed, it becomes less stabilized by its ligaments, but increasingly stabilized by the surrounding muscles as they contract. For coordination exercises, we put all the weight on one foot, with the ipsilateral knee slightly flexed. The positions of arms, head, or trunk can be varied.

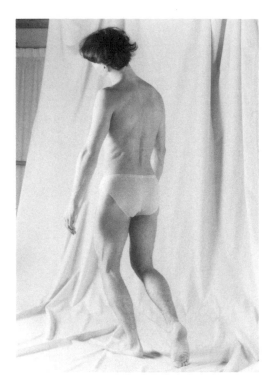

LATERAL MOVEMENTS

Keep your balance on one foot while:

- tilting the head
  to the right or left

- lifting the right
  or left arm

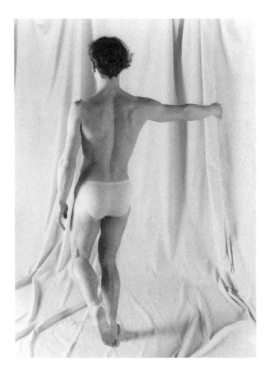

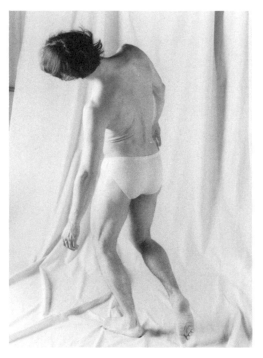

- bending the trunk
  to the right or left.

ROTATION MOVEMENTS

These require constant "rotational rebalancing":

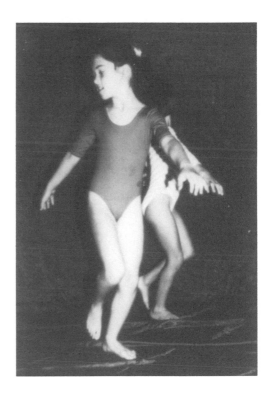

- Turn the head
to the right or left.

- Wave the arms in
circumduction and
rotate the torso on
the pelvis.

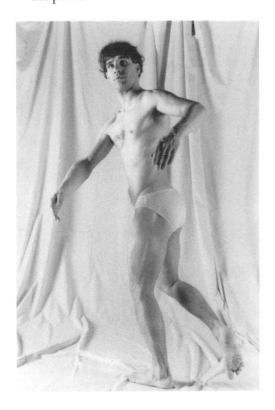

- Add lateral flexion
of the trunk.

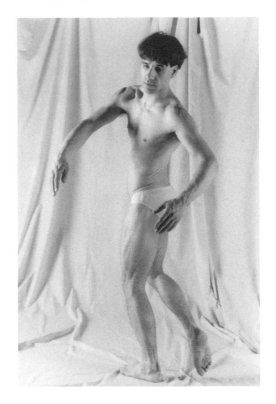

To increase difficulty, close your eyes or
speed up the movement.

Avoid fatigue of the knee cartilages by
changing from one foot to the other
every few minutes.

You can make these coordination
movements more complex and add
variations of your own design.

CHAPTER EIGHT

The Ankle & Foot

. . . .

The foot provides the interface between the human body and the ground which supports it. The structure and function of the foot represent a difficult compromise between strength and flexibility. The ankle is the joint where the vertical plane of the body meets the horizontal plane of the foot. The talus (ankle bone) has the interesting property that no muscles attach to it. Together, the ankle and foot contain 26 bones, 31 joints, and 20 intrinsic muscles, which must contend with the constant force of gravity plus a variety of severe stresses from running, jumping, etc. For most of us, the foot does its job successfully throughout our lives. It should be appreciated as a masterpiece of engineering.

Movements

The ankle is essentially a hinge joint, with the talus being tightly clasped by the lateral and medial malleoli of the fibula and tibia, and the distal end of the tibia. Thus, movement of the talus relative to the tibia and fibula occurs mainly in a sagittal plane (see *AOM*, pp. 244–45).

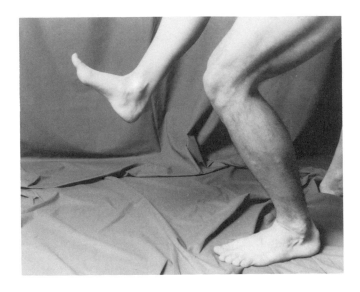

In **dorsiflexion** the dorsal (superior) surface of the foot and the anterior surface of the leg move closer together, i.e., the angle between these two surfaces decreases.

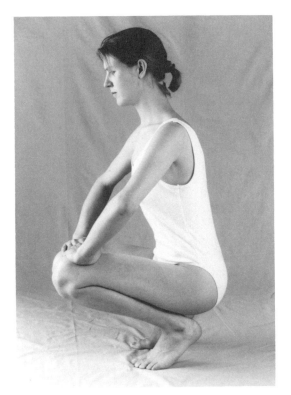

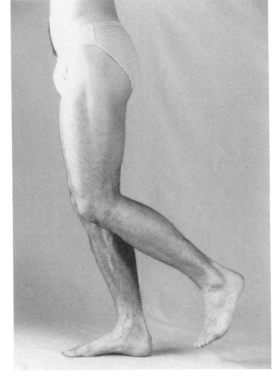

We see this in weight-bearing situations such as squatting, landing from a jump, and supporting the body in a plié.

Non-weight-bearing dorsiflexion occurs when the foot is off the ground about to step forward, climbing stairs, etc.

In **plantar flexion**, or **extension**, the angle between the dorsal surface of the foot and the anterior surface of the leg increases.

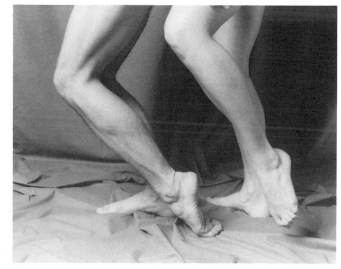

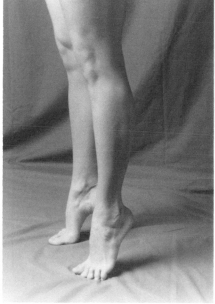

Examples of this movement in weight-bearing are standing on tip-toe . . .

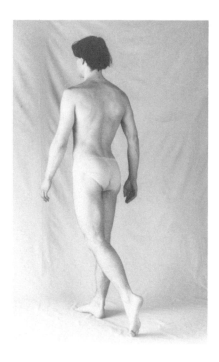

. . . and sitting on the heels.

A non-weight-bearing example is just before the posterior foot leaves the floor in walking.

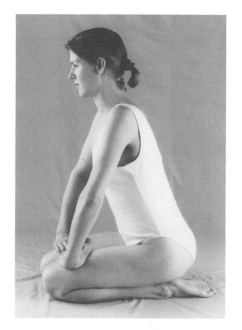

Dorsiflexion and plantar flexion occur mainly where the superior talus meets the tibia/fibula, but also to a minor degree at the joint between the inferior talus and calcaneus (talocalcaneal joint) and more distal joints between the various foot bones.

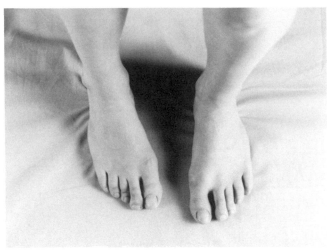

Abduction and adduction of the foot, movements in which the toes move laterally or medially, involve the talocalcaneal and more distal joints rather than the ankle joint.

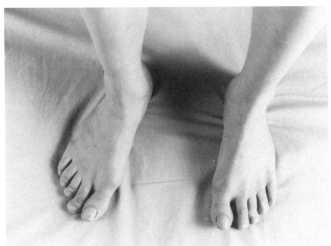

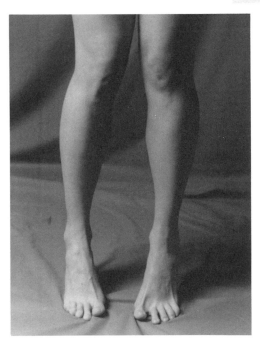

They are easily confused with rotations of the hip or knee joints (see *AOM*, p. 256). They are rare in non-weight-bearing situations, but can be observed when the leg rotates on one weight-bearing foot, or when you stand with your heels off the ground.

In the combination movements called **inversion** and **eversion,** the sole of the foot moves respectively toward and away from the median plane.

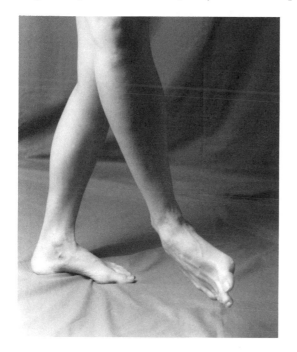

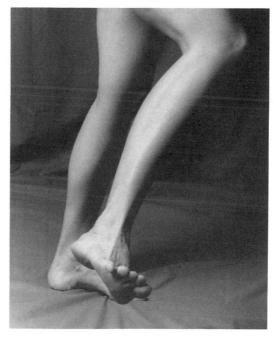

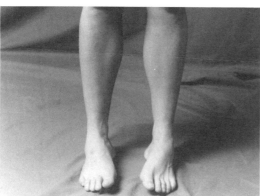

In weight-bearing situations, inversion puts the weight of the body on the lateral edges of the feet,

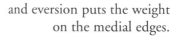

and eversion puts the weight on the medial edges.

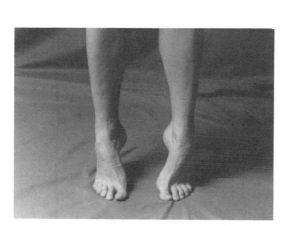

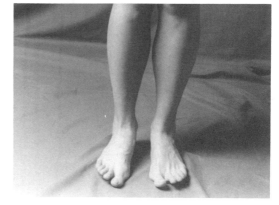

Inversion can be viewed as a combination of plantar flexion and adduction (left), and eversion as a combination of dorsiflexion and abduction (see *AOM*, p. 256).

Flexibility of the ankle

Bony flexibility

The superior talus is wider anteriorly than it is posteriorly. In dorsiflexion, the wide anterior part is firmly held between the two malleoli, and no movement is possible except in a sagittal plane (see *AOM*, pp. 244–45).

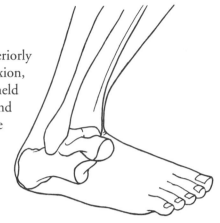

However, in plantar flexion the narrower posterior part is between the malleoli, and limited rotational and lateral movement is theoretically possible.

Thus, the ankle joint is relatively unstable in weight-bearing situations involving plantar flexion, and relies on surrounding ligaments and muscles for reinforcement of the bony structure.

Ligamentary flexibility

The deltoid ligament on the medial side of the ankle is larger and stronger than the three ligaments on the lateral side (see *AOM*, pp. 245–46). Thus, the lateral side is more susceptible to strains or sprains. You should avoid excessive inversion movements which stress the lateral ligaments, e.g., crossing the foot over the opposite thigh without sufficient lateral rotation of the hip joint.

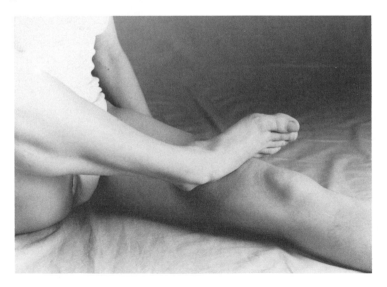

Muscular flexibility

Muscular braking of ankle dorsiflexion is provided by the **gastrocnemius** and **soleus** ("triceps surae"). Recall that gastrocnemius originates on the posterior femur and inserts on calcaneus (see *AOM*, p. 230) and therefore crosses both the knee and ankle joints. Soleus originates on the tibia and fibula and crosses only the ankle joint (see *AOM*, p. 264). These muscles insert onto calcaneus via the common **Achilles tendon**.

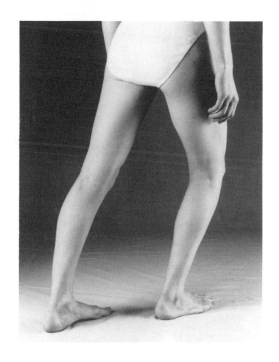

In this photo, on the left leg, gastrocnemius and soleus are completely stretched. On the right leg, soleus is equally stretched (because the ankle is in the same position) but gastrocnemius is not (because the knee is flexed).

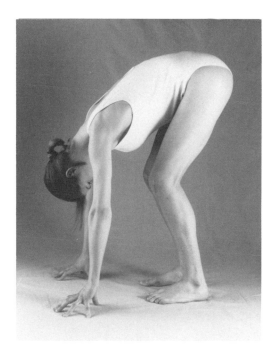

In people who do not exercise much, or women who frequently wear high heels, gastrocnemius and soleus are typically too short. If such people try to bend forward and touch their hands to the floor, you will observe flexion of the knees . . .

. . . and/or lifting of the heels off the floor.

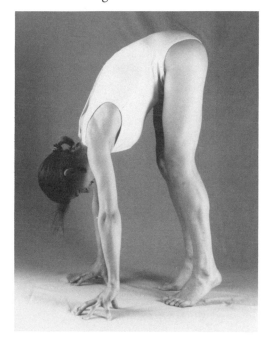

Exercises aimed at stretching gastrocnemius and soleus should always be done in a very gradual, progressive manner. The Achilles tendon, despite being the thickest tendon in the body, is frequently ruptured, especially by sudden and unaccustomed exertion.

Flexibility of the foot

At the **talocalcaneal joint**, talus fits against calcaneus via two (anterior and posterior) articular surfaces (see *AOM*, p. 247). Because of the irregular shapes of the two bones, their oblique orientations, and the two articulating surfaces, there is potential mobility in many directions. However, this mobility is greatly restricted by the presence of the strong interosseus ligament between the two bones and the numerous external ankle ligaments originating from the malleoli (see *AOM*, pp. 245–46). Flexibility at this joint is also restricted by contraction of gastrocnemius, soleus, and various anterior ankle muscles (see *AOM*, p. 257).

Between talus and calcaneus (the "posterior tarsals") and the metatarsal bones are five "anterior tarsals" consisting of cuboid, navicular, and three cuneiforms (see *AOM*, p. 241). The joints of the anterior tarsals are known collectively as the **transverse tarsal joint** and the **cuneiform joints** (see *AOM*, pp. 250–51). The articular planes here are mostly vertical, whereas the plane of the talocalcaneal joint is mostly horizontal. Rotation, abduction, and adduction predominate over plantar flexion and dorsiflexion in the joints of the anterior tarsals. There are numerous ligaments and muscles in this area which restrict movement.

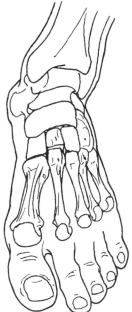

The **tarsometatarsal joints** form an irregular boundary between the cuboid, cuneiforms, and the proximal ends of the five metatarsals (see *AOM*, p. 252). Limited plantar and dorsiflexion is possible at these joints.

The **metatarsophalangeal joints** potentially allow plantar/dorsiflexion, abduction/adduction, and some rotation (see *AOM*, p. 253). However, because most people in the developed world wear shoes and seldom walk barefoot on uneven ground, there is little opportunity for these movements (except for dorsiflexion) to be practiced. Dorsiflexion at the metatarsophalangeal joints (as in running or standing on tiptoe) is common, and has greater ROM and stronger associated muscles than plantar flexion.

The **interphalangeal joints** are all hinge joints. The proximal joints allow only plantar flexion, while the distal joints allow both plantar and dorsiflexion (see *AOM*, p. 253). The proximal joints tend to be in plantar flexion most of the time; they should be checked to make sure straight alignment is still possible. Sometimes mobility of the distal joints is lost through inactivity; this should be checked and the mobility recovered if necessary.

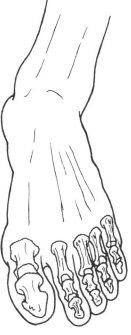

Working the ankle and foot muscles

There are two types of muscles in this area. **Intrinsic muscles** are small ones which originate on other foot or ankle bones and act only on joints within the foot. Because of the inactivity imposed by constant wearing of shoes, intrinsic muscles are often found to be functioning poorly or not at all. **Extrinsic muscles** originate from the tibia, fibula, or femur. They act on the ankle as well as joints within the foot. They are much larger, more powerful, and more frequently used than the intrinsic muscles.

We must therefore consider two very different types of exercises:
- those focused on the intrinsic muscles, involving precise and small movements, designed to recover mobility lost because of shoe wearing
- larger, general exercises for the extrinsic muscles, which can easily and naturally be combined with leg exercises (see "The plié," p. 252).

Extrinsic muscles

The plantar flexors are more numerous and stronger than the dorsiflexors (see *AOM*, p. 271). Why? Because in walking or running it is the propulsion phase—where the posterior foot pushes off from the ground—that requires the most strength. Lifting (dorsiflexion) of the foot as it moves forward after pushing off requires much less strength.

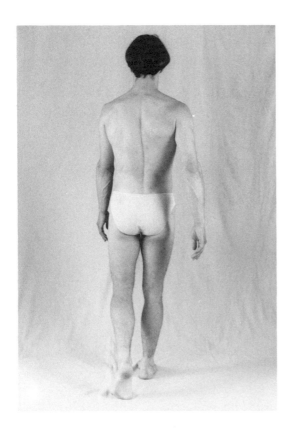
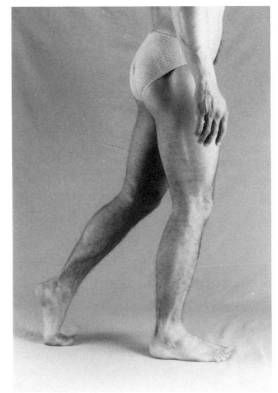

Visualize a longitudinal plane of the foot passing through the center of the talus and the second toe. The muscles whose tendons run medial to this plane are the invertors/adductors, while those whose tendons run lateral to the plane are the evertors/abductors. The former group are more numerous and stronger than the latter group (see *AOM*, p. 271). Why? Because the foot is built like a vault whose medial arch is more prominent and more involved in propulsion than the lateral arch (see *AOM*, pp. 273–74). The medial arch is maintained not by stacking of bones, but by the presence of strong ligaments and tendons.

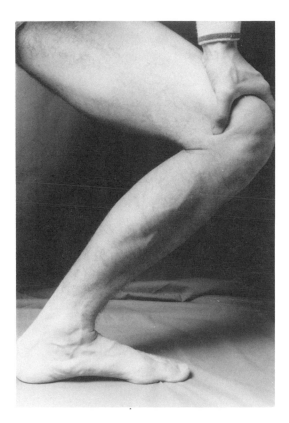

The medial arch can change its shape. It becomes somewhat flattened during weight-bearing dorsiflexion . . .

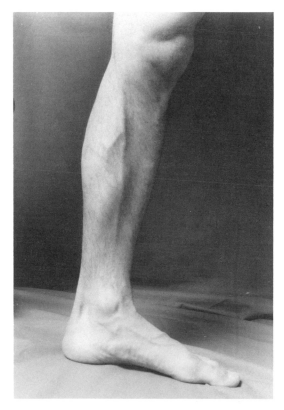

. . . and returns to normal during rest. We often see people invert their feet when standing for a long time; this has the effect of resting the invertor/adductor muscles which support the medial arch.

Coordination of the ankle and foot

It is interesting to consider, on one hand, how the ankle is stabilized by the interplay of muscles, and, on the other hand, how its positioning affects the positioning of more distal foot joints, leading to different ways of "forming" the foot.

Ankle joint

As explained above and in *AOM* (pp. 244–45, 272), the bony structure of the ankle is more stable in dorsiflexion than in plantar flexion. Also, in plantar flexion the medial ankle ligaments are taut anteriorly and slack posteriorly. Therefore, in this position there is greater risk of "wrong" movement at the ankle (twisting of the talus in inversion) and of sprains, particularly of the anterior talofibular ligament (see *AOM*, p. 246). The instability associated with plantar flexion is compensated for by contraction of four muscles which pull down the fibula (and its lateral malleolus) and tighten the "pincer" formed by the two malleoli around the talus (see *AOM*, p. 272).

This happens only in active dorsiflexion, e.g., standing on tiptoe. Exercises for the muscles involved in this type of coordination are presented on pp. 258–59.

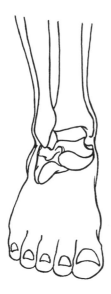

Orientation of the talus is affected by the positions of the tibia and fibula. Recall that there are conditions "genu valgum" and "genu varum" (see p. 186) in which the knees in standing position are located more medially or laterally than average. If the leg bones are leaning laterally or medially, they will tend to tilt the talus in the same direction.

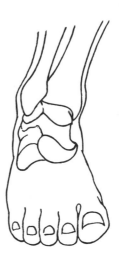

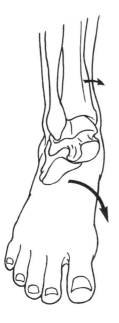

Likewise, medial rotation at the knee causes the lateral (fibular) malleolus to push the talus in medial rotation and evert the foot at the talocalcaneal joint.

Lateral rotation at the knee causes the medial malleolus to push the talus in lateral rotation and invert the foot at the talocalcaneal joint.

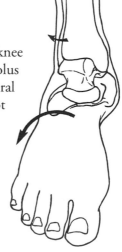

Orientation of the leg bones and talus always affects the orientation and shape of the anterior foot, but details of this relationship vary among individuals.

Talocalcaneal joint

As mentioned above, the unusual shape and orientation of the talus and calcaneus give this joint potential mobility in many directions. No muscles attach on talus. Its movement depends mostly on what the surrounding bones are doing. The only muscles inserting on calcaneus are gastrocnemius and soleus, via their common Achilles tendon. However, several muscles with more anterior insertions run alongside calcaneus and are able to push it to one side or the other.

Orientation of the talocalcaneal joint is dictated by the balance and orientation of the anterior foot, and by distribution of body weight. Viewed from behind, the calf, Achilles tendon, and calcaneus form a shape something like an hourglass.

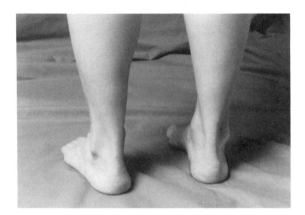

When body weight is directed straight downward at the center of the heel, the Achilles tendon and "hourglass" are vertical.

When weight falls on the inside, the foot tends to evert and the "hourglass" leans medially.

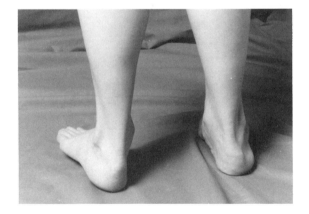

When weight falls to the outside, the foot inverts and the "hourglass" leans laterally.

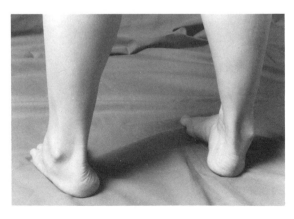

Transverse tarsal joint

This joint is oriented vertically whereas the joints above it (talocalcaneal, ankle, knee) are essentially horizontal. The foot can be viewed as a tripod with weight directed to three points: the heel, and the heads of metatarsals I and V. By torsion (twisting), the transverse tarsal joint can shift weight to either metatarsal I or V, or balance between them.

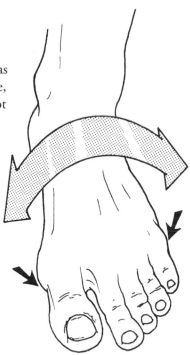

Torsion results from interplay between extrinsic and intrinsic muscle contractions and distribution of body weight. In addition, the big toe can take some weight, thereby "freeing" the head of metatarsal I.

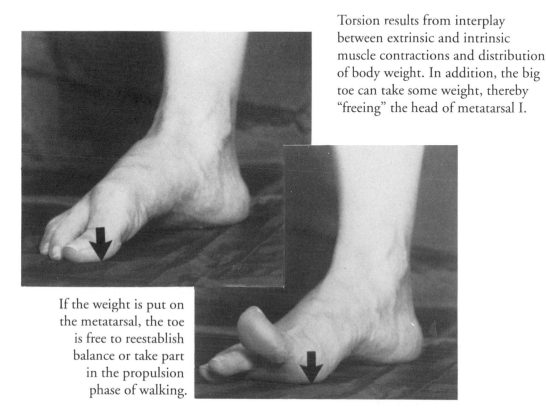

If the weight is put on the metatarsal, the toe is free to reestablish balance or take part in the propulsion phase of walking.

Coordination in weight-bearing situations

The three corners of the foot "tripod" described above also form the endpoints of the three arches: the medial arch, lateral arch (which cannot be seen externally), and anterior arch. Recall that the three arches are sustained by action of the numerous intrinsic muscles and ligaments. It is interesting to observe what happens to the tripod in response to changing body weight distribution.

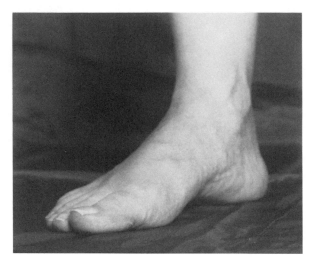

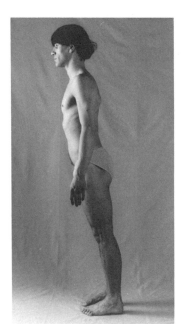

As the body tilts forward, weight is directed to the two anterior corners of the tripod (metatarsal I and V heads) and removed from the heel, and the toes "grip" (plantar flexion).

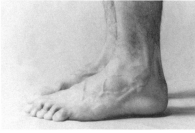

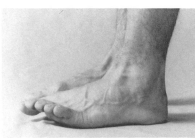

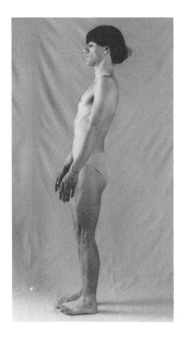

As the body tilts backward, weight is directed onto the heel and removed from the metatarsal heads, and the toes dorsiflex.

Try experiencing some weight-bearing situations between these two extremes.

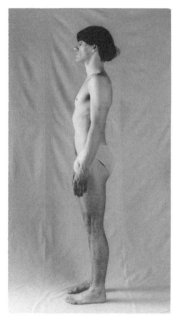

Seventy-five percent of the weight on the heel, twenty-five percent on the metatarsals (none on the toes). This position helps rest the arch-sustaining muscles because calcaneus is bearing most of the weight. Tibia is essentially balanced on top of talus, requiring only minimal muscular contractions. This is a good position to adopt when standing for long periods of time because of the small muscular effort required.

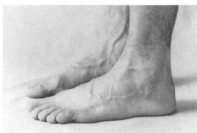

Balance, however, is precarious; you are on the verge of falling backward. Constant, tiny proprioceptive adjustments of the talocalcaneal and other foot joints are required.

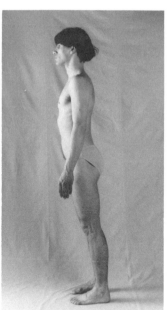

Fifty percent of the weight on the heel, fifty percent on the metatarsals. The arches are bearing much of the body weight here, and all the arch-sustaining muscles are contracting. Tibia is not vertical and not balanced on talus. Gastrocnemius and soleus are contracting to maintain or recover balance. Fine proprioceptive adjustments of the talocalcaneal joint are not required. Balance is easier; there is a "margin of error" for leaning farther forward or backward, regulated by less or more contraction of gastrocnemius. This is not a resting position but rather a "ready" position prior to initiation of movement.

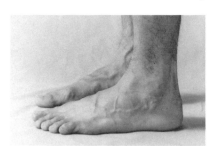

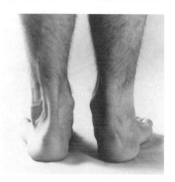

Sideways leaning. Weight is disproportionately directed to the medial or lateral edge of the foot. This is particularly evident when one foot is raised off the ground.

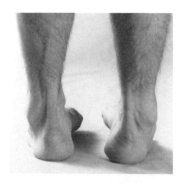

Practice pages: Ankle and foot

Mobilizing the ankle

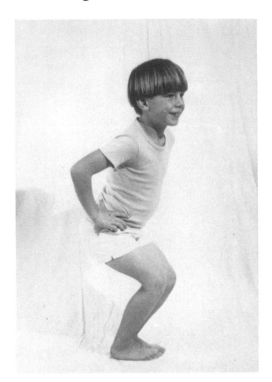

DORSIFLEXION

This movement is important in cushioning the landing phase of a jump. In the "demi-plié" (half bent) position, the hips and knees are flexed and the heels remain in contact with the floor. You can lean on a bar to take some weight off the ankle.

Squatting with feet together strongly dorsiflexes the ankle. It is important to keep both heels on the floor. To maintain your balance in this position, you must direct much of the body's weight to the anterior foot. This requires maximum ROM in flexion at the hip, knee, and ankle joints.

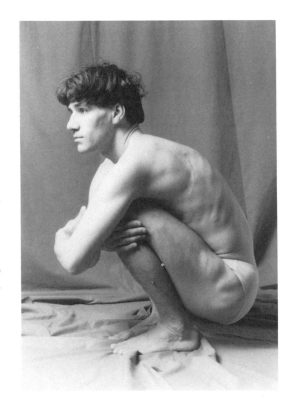

If ROM is inadequate at one or more of these joints, balancing is very difficult and you will tend to fall backward. There are two ways to compensate:

- Raise the heels, transfer weight to the anterior foot, and balance (precariously) on the toes. Since the ankle is no longer being dorsiflexed, this position is useless for our purposes.

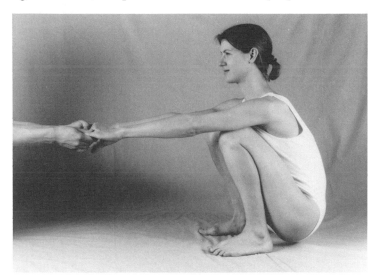

- Hold onto some anchoring point in front of you (a bar or partner).

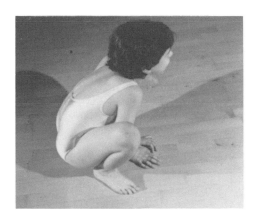

Do not confuse this with the limbering exercise for the hip (p. 158), where the knees are spread apart and the trunk held between them. This latter position requires good ROM at the hip, but not so much at the ankle.

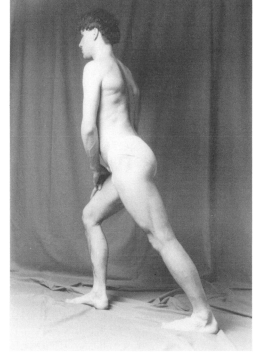

If you don't like squatting, you can dorsiflex one ankle at a time by standing in the position shown. You can take some weight off the stretched (posterior) ankle by leaning on a bar or putting your hands on the anterior knee. This is the same position often used for stretching the hamstrings, since the knee is extended.

PLANTAR FLEXION

Very flexible individuals can achieve this by sitting on the heels, with toes straight.

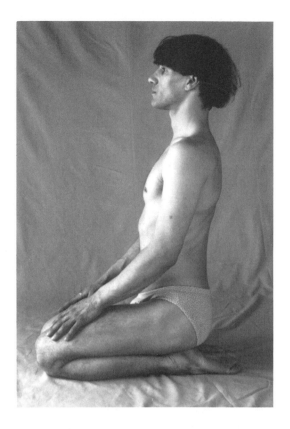

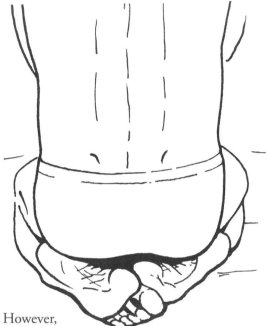

However, many people find this position impossible. The feet may tend to invert and the buttocks rest on the medial arches rather than on the heels.

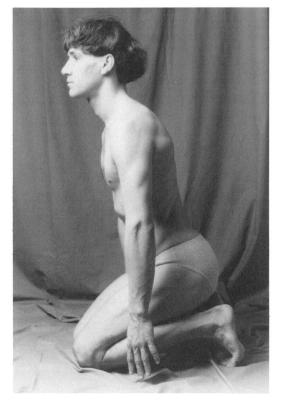

Alternatively, the ankles and toes may end up in dorsiflexion.

An easier approach is to hold the head and shoulders forward, hands placed on the floor on either side of the knees. Start with much of the body weight on the hands, then gradually transfer it to the knees and then the feet. Besides plantar-flexing the ankles, this will stretch the small joints of the feet and the anterior leg muscles which insert on the foot.

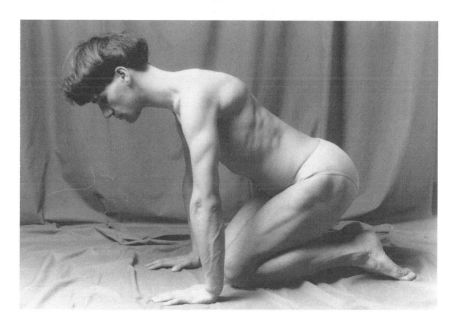

For people who have mastered the "sitting on the heels" position, plantar flexion of the ankle and anterior foot can by increased even more by placing the hands on the floor behind the feet, putting some weight on them, and raising the knees off the floor.

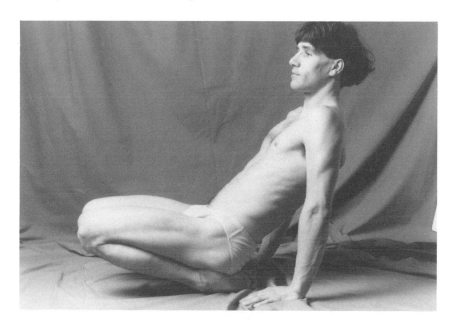

Mobilizing the talocalcaneal joint

Sit down, one leg stretched forward, calcaneus on the floor. Visualize the joint between talus and calcaneus, and try mobilizing it forward and backward. The heel should stay on the floor and the ankle joint move as little as possible. You should feel a sensation as if trying to enlarge or shrink the foot. You can practice this same exercise while standing up or walking slowly.

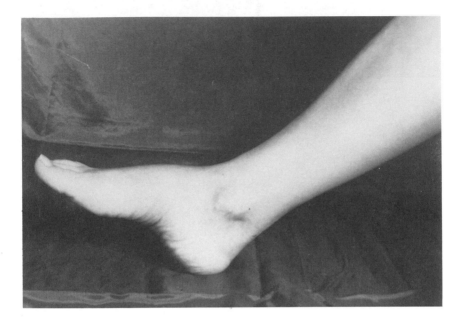

Alternatively, in the seated position, visualize calcaneus as a ball which is pivoting (and the anterior foot with it) on talus.

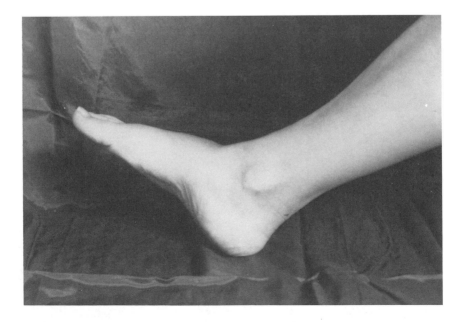

Stand with knees slightly bent so that the Achilles tendons are visible. Simultaneously move both calcaneus bones sideways such that they move away from or toward each other. Make sure the knees do not move. You can put both hands on the knees to ensure that the movement is not originating there.

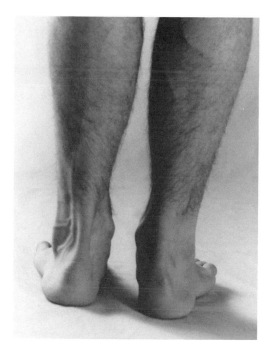 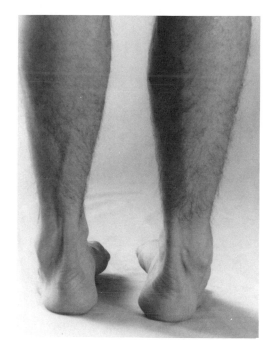

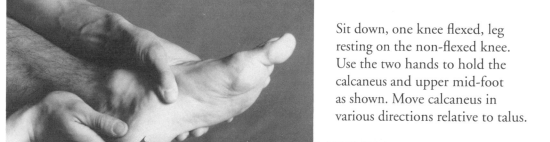

Sit down, one knee flexed, leg resting on the non-flexed knee. Use the two hands to hold the calcaneus and upper mid-foot as shown. Move calcaneus in various directions relative to talus.

Mobilizing the distal joints

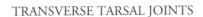

TRANSVERSE TARSAL JOINTS

Sit on the floor. Use one hand to
grip calcaneus, keeping the ankle
joint in fixed dorsiflexion. Hold the
mid-foot with the other hand and
twist it in different directions: medial,
lateral, dorsiflexion, plantar flexion.
Movement should be occurring at the
transverse tarsal joints, not the ankle.

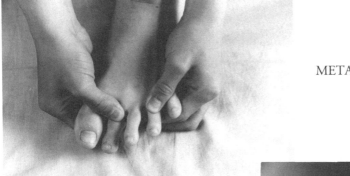

METATARSOPHALANGEALS

These joints can potentially move
in many directions, but some of
their mobility (e.g., plantar flexion)
is frequently lost from prolonged
shoe wearing. Use your hands to
move the first phalanges (not just
the second and third) upward,
downward, and side to side. Try to
keep the metatarsals relatively fixed.

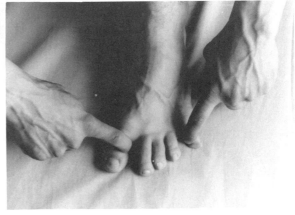

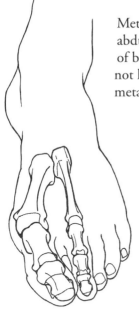

Metatarsophalangeal joint I sometimes appears to be stiffened in abduction, i.e., the big toe is pressed against the second toe instead of being straight. Trying to adduct the big toe by pulling on it is usually not helpful because the problem originates more proximally: the head of metatarsal I is directed medially, too far from the head of metatarsal II.

Start by using one hand to squeeze the metatarsals firmly together such that I is brought closer to II.

Then, use the other hand to move the big toe gently in various directions, with the objective of improving or regaining capsular mobility.

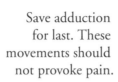

Save adduction for last. These movements should not provoke pain.

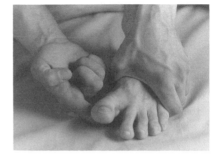

INTERPHALANGEALS

These are hinge joints. Use the hands to gently mobilize them. Make sure the proximal joints can straighten out, and are not stiffened in plantar flexion. Remember the distal joints can dorsiflex as well as plantar flex.

Muscle strengthening: Intrinsic

INTEROSSEI (see *AOM*, pp. 266–67)

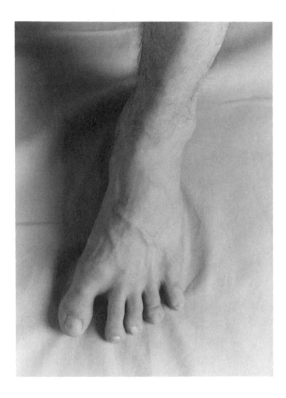

Start by using them as abductors
and adductors: spread the toes
apart and squeeze them together.
These muscles can bring the
metatarsals closer together,
as well as the phalanges.

The interossei can also plantar flex the metatarsophalangeal joints and straighten out the
proximal interphalangeals.

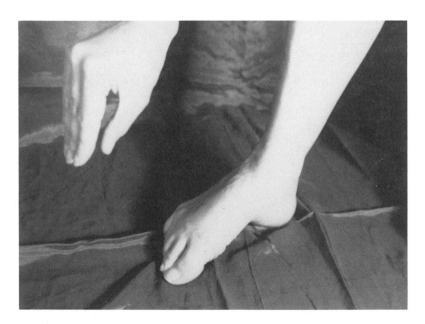

This movement is easily confused with plantar flexion of the proximal interphalangeals, the action of flexor digitorum longus (see *AOM*, p. 262).

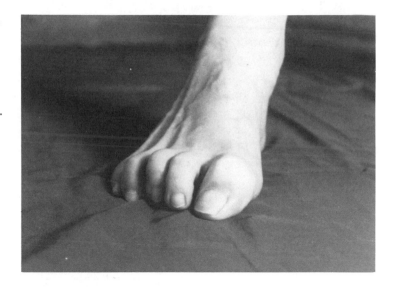

If you find it difficult, approach it by a two-step process:

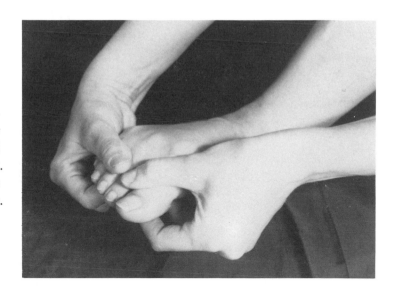

- Move the metatarso-phalangeals passively with your hand and feel the plantar flexion. Make the heads of the metatarsals protrude.

- Practice the movement with your hand (see photo on opposite page) and make the foot mimic the hand.

Once you have mastered the movement, increase the work of the muscles by leaning on the toes. You may feel the contraction of the interossei as a cramping sensation between the metatarsals.

ABDUCTOR HALLUCIS (see *AOM*, p. 269)

This large intrinsic muscle contributes to the medial arch of the foot. Abducting the big toe (moving it medially away from the other toes) is easy for barefoot babies, but difficult for most adults. We are unaccustomed to giving the neuromotor command. There may also be some stiffening of the joint.

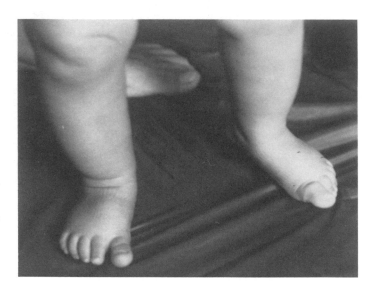

Start with passive movement. Use one hand to immobilize the metatarsals, and the other to abduct the toe.

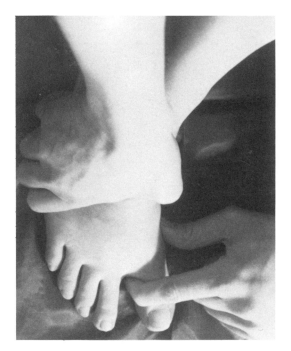

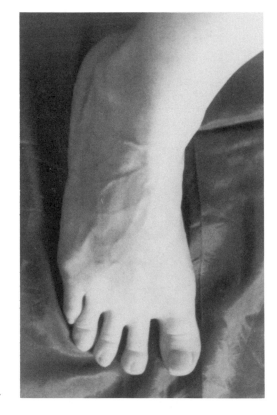

As you become used to the feeling, gradually shift from passive to active movement.

FLEXOR HALLUCIS BREVIS (see *AOM*, p. 269)

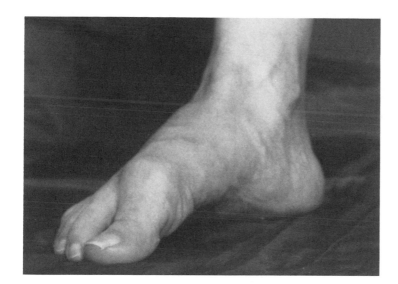

This is a plantar flexor of proximal phalanx I. Distribute your weight evenly along the foot, then press the big toe against the floor.

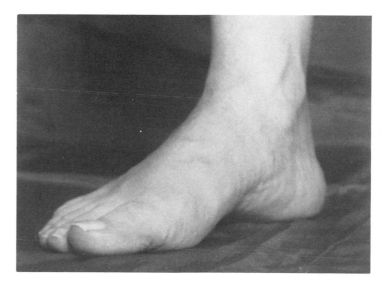

This is not to be confused with putting your weight on the head of metatarsal I (see p. 222).

LATERAL MUSCLES

Abductor digiti minimi and flexor digiti minimi brevis (see *AOM*, p. 270) move the little toe and contribute to the lateral arch of the foot. If you have difficulty activating these muscles, try the same approach as for abductor hallucis: immobilize the metatarsals, start with passive movements using the other hand, then gradually shift to active movement of the little toe in various directions.

Muscle strengthening: Extrinsic

These large muscles should each be exercised in isolation from the others. Familiar combination movements such as walking tend to work some extrinsic muscles more than others.

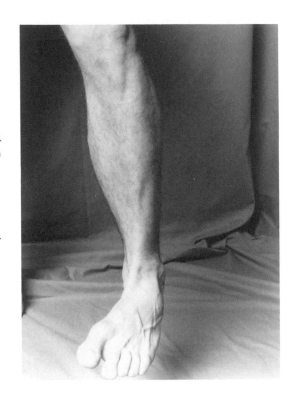

TIBIALIS ANTERIOR
(see *AOM*, p. 258)

Invert the foot. You will
see the body of this muscle
contracting at the upper tibia.

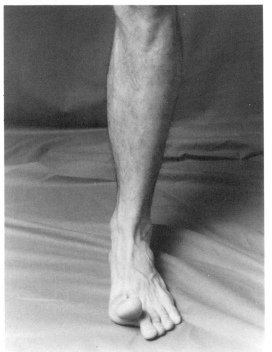

EXTENSOR HALLUCIS LONGUS
(see *AOM*, p. 258)

Dorsiflex the big toe.
Try to keep the other
toes relaxed.

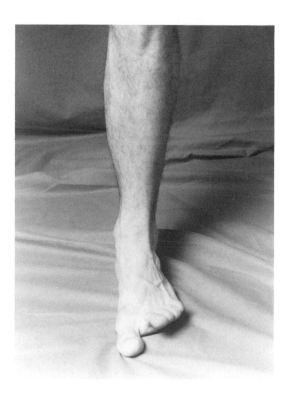

EXTENSOR DIGITORUM LONGUS
(see *AOM*, p. 259)

Dorsiflex toes II through V but try to keep
the big toe relaxed. Once you have mastered
this, try more difficult variations:
- Dorsiflex toes II through V in sequence,
  then in reverse sequence, as if playing
  scales on the piano.
- Take turns exercising extensor hallucis
  longus and extensor digitorum longus;
  lift the big toe, then the other four.

For the three exercises above, keep
your body weight mostly on calcaneus.
If the weight is too far forward, there will be
a tendency to grip (plantar flex) the toes.

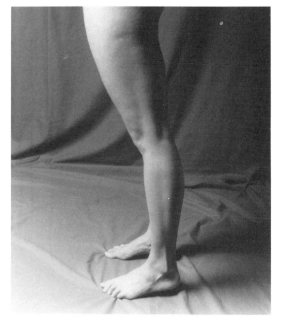

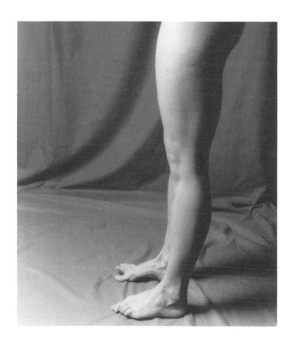

As your weight shifts posteriorly,
the above three muscles contract
together to reestablish balance, and
you can see their tendons protruding
in front of the ankle.

PERONEUS BREVIS AND PERONEUS LONGUS (see *AOM*, p. 260)

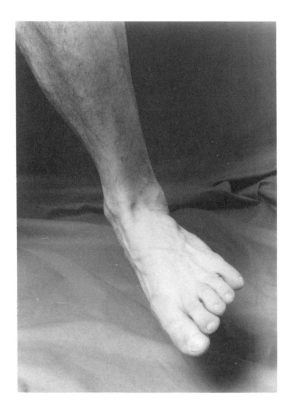

Evert the foot. Move it in a circular fashion while it is everted, and try wrinkling the lateral edge.

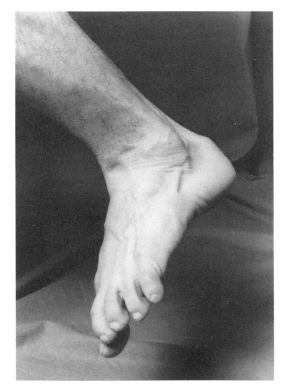

These two muscles have their bodies next to the fibula, where you can see them contract as you stand on tiptoe or balance on one foot.

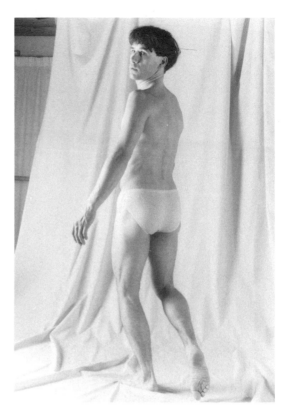

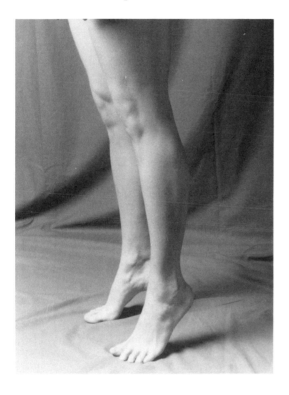

They both contribute to the lateral (weight-bearing) arch of the foot. The tendons of peroneus longus and tibialis posterior cross on the underside of the foot, forming a "sling" which helps keep the mid-foot elevated (see *AOM*, p. 261).

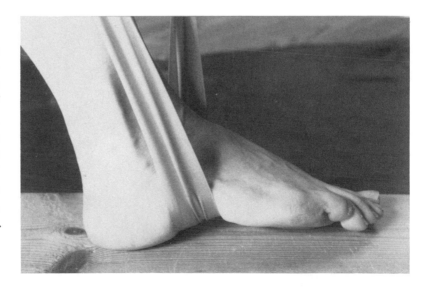

FLEXOR HALLUCIS LONGUS (see *AOM*, p. 263)

This is a plantar flexor of the big toe, like flexor hallucis brevis, but it is extrinsic (originating from fibula) and inserts on the distal rather than proximal phalanx. The exercise is the same: press the big toe against the floor without putting extra weight on the head of metatarsal I. This muscle crosses several joints and is important in coordinating the action of the foot and ankle:

- It "pulls" the tibia and fibula closer together.
- It stabilizes the talus posteriorly (its tendon is the only one that slides on the talus; see *AOM*, p. 240).
- It supports the medial arch.

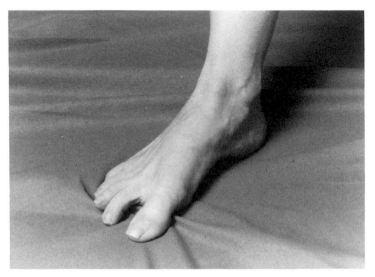

FLEXOR DIGITORUM LONGUS (see *AOM*, p. 262)

This is the major plantar flexor of toes II through V. Press these toes (not the big toe) against the floor, with body weight evenly distributed along the foot (metatarsal heads are neither pressed down nor lifted). For more difficulty, try pressing toes II through V in sequence, then reverse sequence.

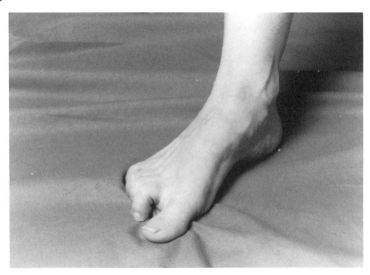

TIBIALIS POSTERIOR (see *AOM*, p. 262)

As mentioned above, the tendons of this muscle and peroneus longus form an X-shaped "sling" on the underside of the foot which helps maintain the arched shape.

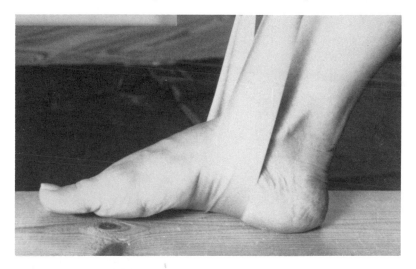

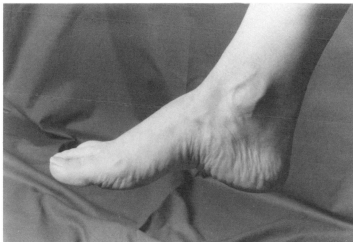

It is difficult to isolate contraction of tibialis posterior, the deepest calf muscle. Keeping the ankle fixed, try to arch the foot more than usual:

• with contraction

• without contraction

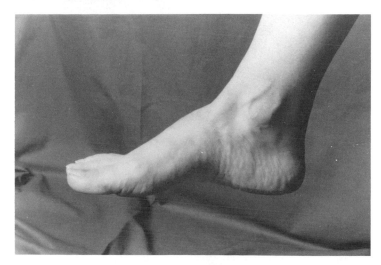

Muscular coordination

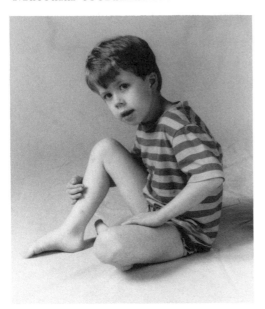

1. Sit on the floor, one flexed knee raised, the other near the ground for support.

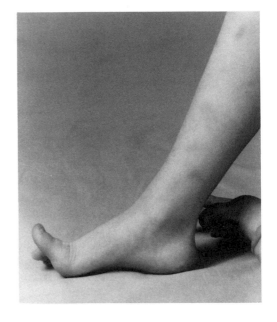

Start with the foot flat, close to the body. Gradually move the foot away with a crawling movement. Keep the heel in contact with the floor, but alternately plantar flex and dorsiflex the toes. Keep the arch high. Bring the foot back toward the body in the same way.

Same exercise but try to keep the extrinsic muscles relaxed (put a hand on the calf to check this). This forces the intrinsic muscles to do more of the work.

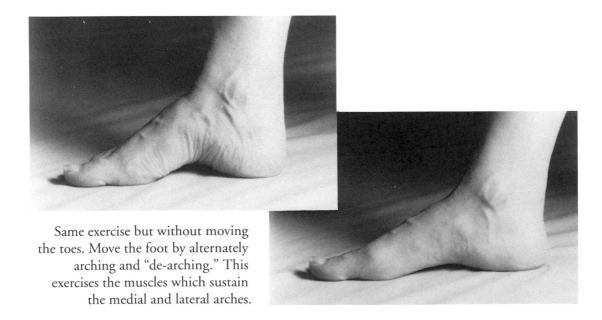

Same exercise but without moving the toes. Move the foot by alternately arching and "de-arching." This exercises the muscles which sustain the medial and lateral arches.

2. Sit on the floor, hips abducted,
heels touching. Arch the feet
and touch the big toes together.

Dorsiflex the toes and touch
the metatarsal I heads together.

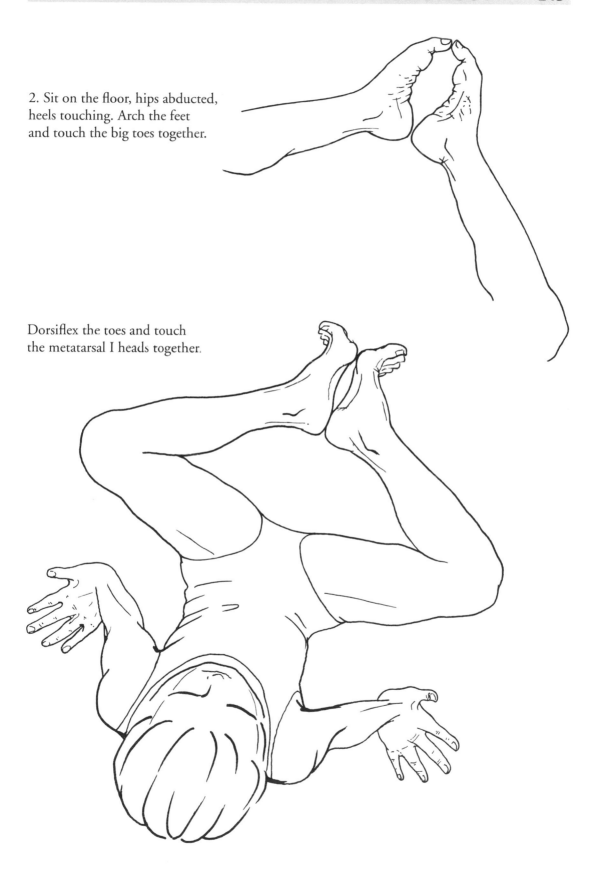

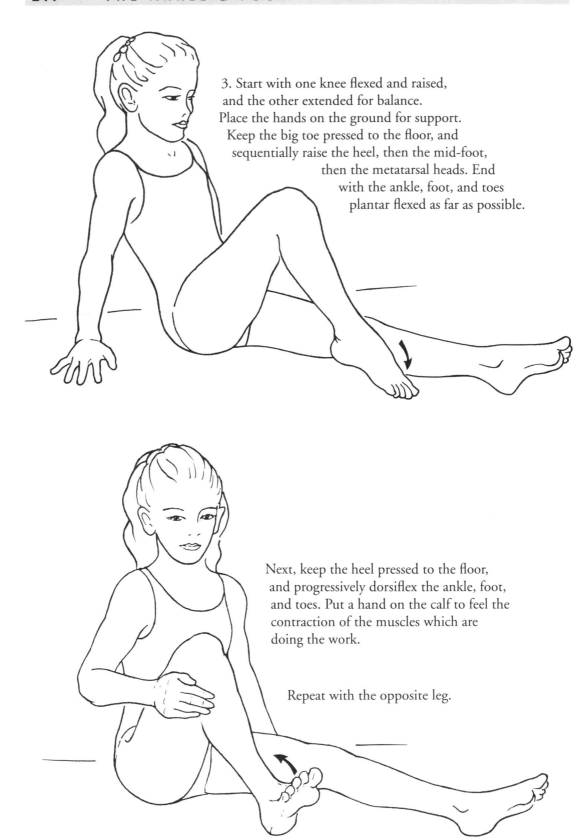

3. Start with one knee flexed and raised,
and the other extended for balance.
Place the hands on the ground for support.
Keep the big toe pressed to the floor, and
sequentially raise the heel, then the mid-foot,
then the metatarsal heads. End
with the ankle, foot, and toes
plantar flexed as far as possible.

Next, keep the heel pressed to the floor,
and progressively dorsiflex the ankle, foot,
and toes. Put a hand on the calf to feel the
contraction of the muscles which are
doing the work.

Repeat with the opposite leg.

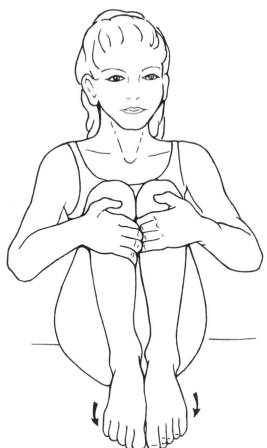

After you've mastered this, do the same exercise with both feet simultaneously. Keep the various parts of the feet "in synch" during the sequential plantar flexion. You can add further coordination and precision by keeping the right and left knees, medial malleoli, and medial edges of the feet in contact throughout.

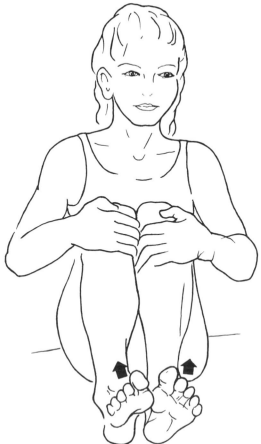

CHAPTER NINE

Coordination of Hip, Knee & Foot

In the preceding chapters we have seen many examples of the interdependence of these joints in terms of body weight distribution, muscle function, and orientation of bones. There are several muscles which span the hip and knee. Gastrocnemius spans the knee and ankle. In this chapter (which consists entirely of "practice pages") we will learn to coordinate movements of these joints, and see how exercises can be "guided" from the top (i.e., hip), from the bottom (i.e., foot), or even from both ends at once.

Guiding from the hip

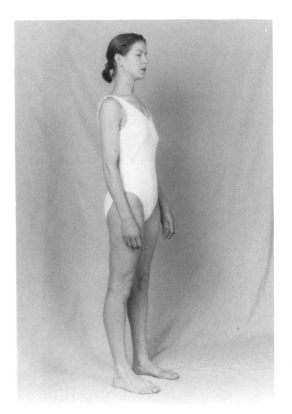

Stand up, knees straight, feet parallel and directly under the hips, weight mostly on the heels. Medially rotate the hips slightly, and observe the consequences distally:

- The patellas move medially to partially "face" each other.

- Posteriorly, the popliteal spaces are directed somewhat laterally.

- The tibias are medially rotated.

- There is some eversion of the posterior feet.

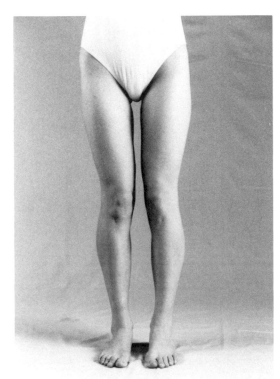

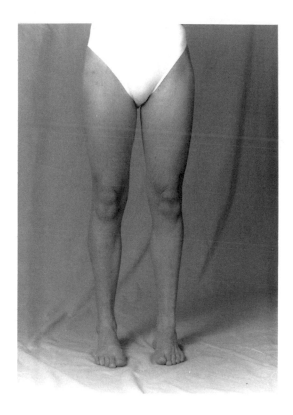

Alternatively, contract the gluteal muscles to laterally rotate the hips. Observe the consequences:

• The patellas face laterally.
• The tibias are laterally rotated.
• The posterior foot is inverted.

You can see how movement at the hip can "guide" the leg and foot.

There is an intermediate position between these two extremes: slight lateral rotation at the hips, but guiding the femurs in such a way that the patellas still face directly forward. Visualize the sacrum being heavy at the back of the pelvis, and this weight guiding the femurs into slight lateral rotation.

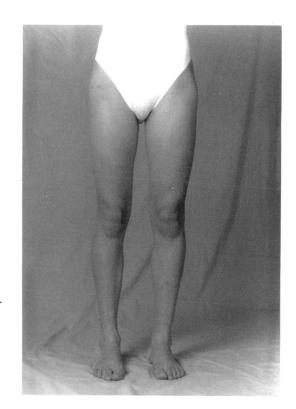

Guiding from the foot

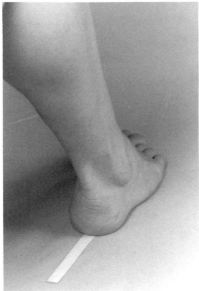

Sit or kneel with one foot flat on the floor.
Press the middle part of the heel against the
floor. Be aware of the median line of the heel,
as if it were the blade of an ice skate.

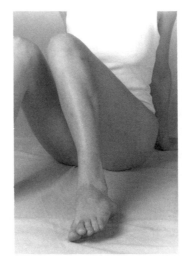 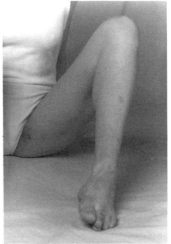

Rotate the hip slightly such
that the knee swings medially
or laterally. The heel will tend
at first to lean to the same side
as the knee. But try to keep pressure on the median line of the heel by actively holding the
calcaneus in place. This is a proprioceptive balancing action of the talocalcaneal joint.

Next, press each point of the foot "tripod" against the floor in succession:

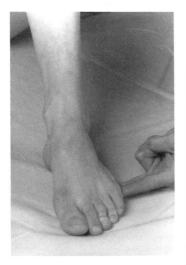

• head of metatarsal V

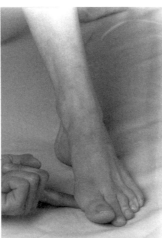

• head of metatarsal I
  (keep the big toe relaxed)

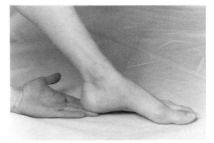

• heel

Find a position in which the three points are pressing down with equal strength (keep the toes relaxed).

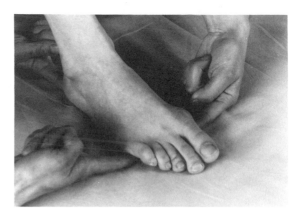

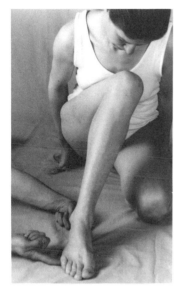

Swing the knee from side to side as before. Observe how the pressure of the tripod shifts in the same direction as the knee. Continue swinging the knee, but try to keep the pressure of the three points constant. Next, try reversing the natural tendency: when the knee moves medially, increase the pressure on the lateral side of the tripod, and vice versa.

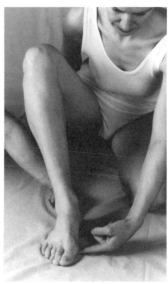

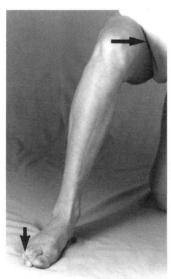

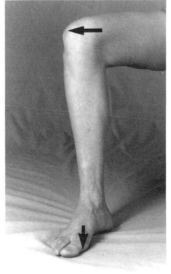

This is tricky. As the knee swings medially, you must not only keep the lateral foot points on the floor, but try to actively push them against the floor. This pushing action will influence the knee and tend to make it move laterally again. Reverse the sequence. Swing the knee laterally, then use pressure on the medial foot points to orient the knee more medially again.

This exercise helps you feel how the foot can, by its selective pressure against the floor, "guide" the leg from the bottom up. This same principle can be applied in weight-bearing situations in all the following exercises.

The plié

In this movement, the trunk moves downward but stays in a vertical orientation. The hips, knees and ankles flex.

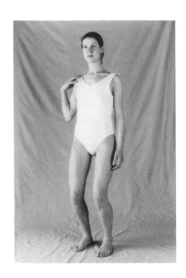

In the "half plié," the heels remain in contact with the floor.

In the "grand plié," the heels come off the floor, knees are fully flexed, and buttocks are lowered close to the feet.

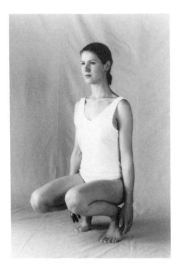

In practicing pliés, we learn to guide the alignment of the femur and tibia. If you are teaching a class, proceed progressively from simple to more difficult movements, as described below.

Feet together

When starting out with pliés, keep the medial malleoli and knees touching. You may notice some "bad" tendencies which need to be eliminated:

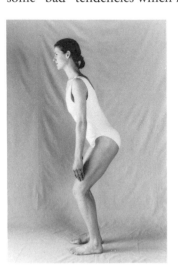

- Sticking out the buttocks. To counter this, imagine that the back is sliding down along a wall, or that you are trying to "sit straight down" above the feet.

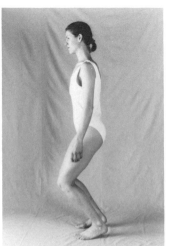

- Raising the heels from the floor.

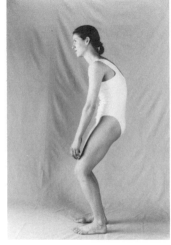

- Rounding the spine. It is very important to keep the spine straight and vertically oriented.

Feet apart

In the next stage, move the feet apart as shown and keep them parallel. A new problem you may encounter is the knees moving closer to each other as the trunk descends. To counteract this:

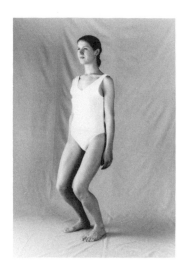

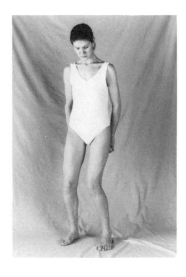

• Place the feet firmly as if on two rails which run from the second toe to the midpoint of the heel. The knees should stay directly above these "rails."

• Imagine that there is a ball occupying the space between the two feet, and another ball of the same size separating the two knees. Again, as the knees are bent they should stay directly above the second toes. The guiding for this orientation comes from the hips.

Become aware of the slight lateral rotation of the femurs and medial rotation of the tibias. It may help to visualize this if you place one hand above the other and turn them in opposite directions, as if wringing a towel. Alternatively, place the hands on the thighs. Slide the hands slightly toward the outside during the descending plié, and toward the inside during the ascending plié.

You can add an arm movement to the descending plié. With arms apart and slightly away from the body, draw a half circle toward the outside which mimics the action of the gluteus maximus.

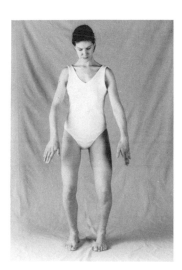

Lateral hip rotation

The feet-together and feet-parallel pliés described above must be mastered before moving on to this more complex stage. You need to understand the basic guiding action in order to maintain precision when adding the lateral rotation ("opening") movement.

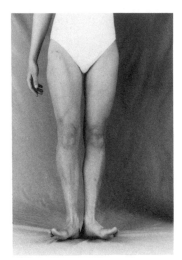

The opening movement should come from the hips only. Start with feet together, then shift the weight to the heels and laterally rotate the hips.

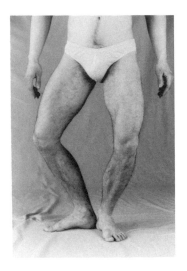

The lower legs form a V shape. Shift the weight more forward on the foot tripod. Do not try to open the V wider than the hips allow you to. For some individuals, the V will be asymmetrical because the two hips have different ROM for lateral rotation. Don't try to "correct" this asymmetry; doing so tends to force undesirable compensations in the pelvis or spine.

Try a similar opening movement with the feet apart. Don't let the knees sag medially; this stretches the medial collateral ligament (see p. 190).

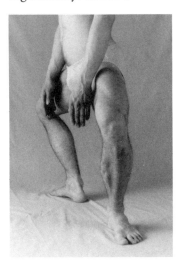

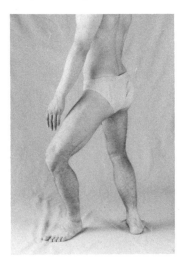

Next, place one foot farther forward, the other behind, while maintaining the opening.

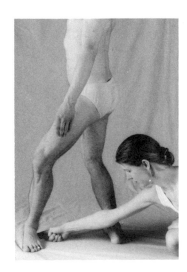

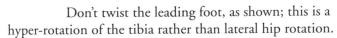

Don't twist the leading foot, as shown; this is a hyper-rotation of the tibia rather than lateral hip rotation.

Lowering and raising actions

For either the plié or grand plié, three key criteria are:
- alignment of the patella above the second toe
- maximum ROM in the opening movement
- keeping the spine straight and vertically oriented while lowering the trunk.

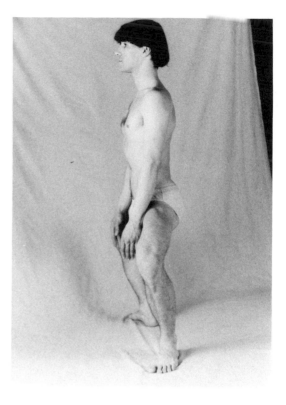

The raising action of the plié is sometimes considered as the "resting" phase, since the lowering action requires greater concentration. Visualize the feet pushing the floor away during the raising action. There is slight medial rotation of the femurs and lateral rotation of the tibias in this phase, the opposite of what happens during lowering.

In a lateral rotation plié, when the knees extend, the hips must remain open. The plié in its movement downward and upward is like an "open book." Progressively, work on coming up more quickly, and link this movement to a raising of the heels. This is a preparatory exercise for the propulsion phase of jumps.

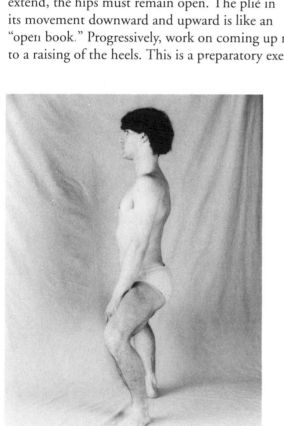

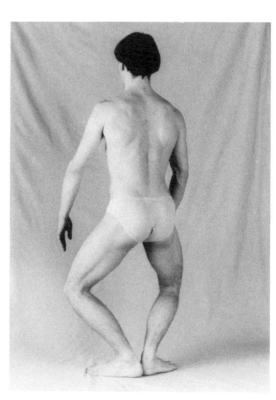

Swinging movements

Here, you shift the weight of the body from one foot to the other, knees slightly flexed. This is different from shifting of the weight during walking.

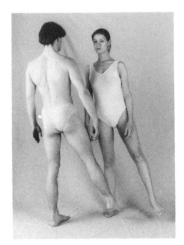

SIDEWAYS SWINGING

This is the easier, "beginning" movement. Stand with feet parallel. Shift all the weight to one foot and bend that knee. Place the other foot down and slightly to the side, plié, then shift the weight to this foot.

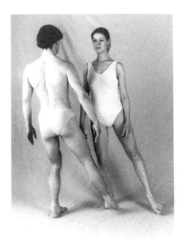

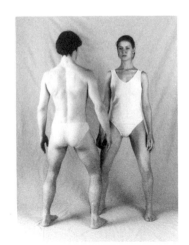

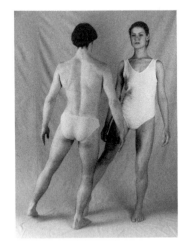

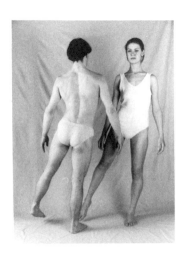

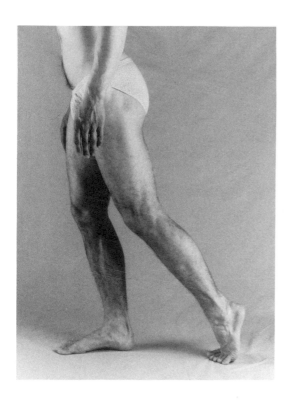

FRONT TO BACK SWINGING

Similar to above, but with a different direction of movement. Be sure the trunk stays vertical and straight. There is often a tendency to either protrude the buttocks or move the trunk forward by hip flexion.

For the leg receiving the weight:
• The foot "unrolls" from front to back.
• Patella should stay above the second toe.
• Balance the body weight on the foot tripod.

For the leg leaving the floor, the parts of the foot are lifted in the following order:
• heel
• lateral arch
• medial arch
• toes.

Next, try swinging with the hips in open position. The lateral rotation causes the knee and foot to lose their "landmarks." Make sure that the rotation really comes from the hip, and guide the leg from the hip as shown on pp. 248–49.

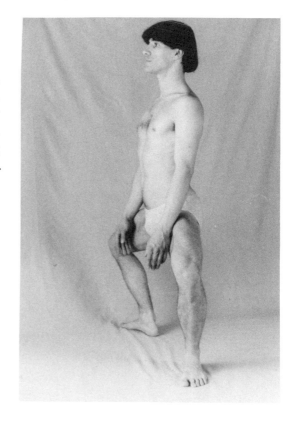

For increased difficulty, try these exercises with eyes closed, or put most of the weight on the anterior foot and less on the heels.

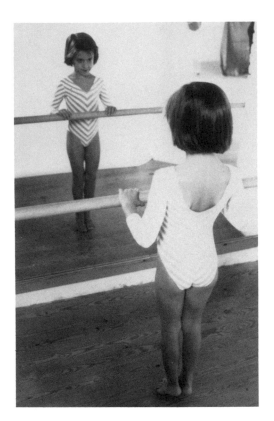

Standing on the toes*

Like the plié, this is an essential movement for ballet dancers, and is practiced in every class, with progression from simple to more difficult variations. At first, use a bar or other support to help with balance.

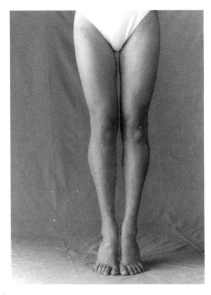

With feet together, raise the heels, pressing the metatarsal heads against the floor. Body weight is evenly distributed along the axis of the second toe. There is practically no weight on the fifth toe.

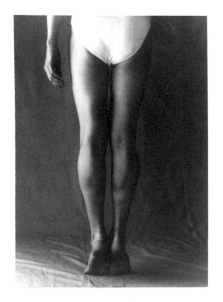

Keep the two medial malleoli in contact with each other. This prevents the feet from going into inversion.

Feel the tightening of the tibia and fibula together, from a deep muscular contraction located just behind them (not to be confused with the more superficial contraction of the gastrocnemius and soleus). This deep contraction runs obliquely, from under the lateral knee toward the medial malleolus. Also feel the precise positioning and "locking" of the talus between the two malleoli (see p. 218).

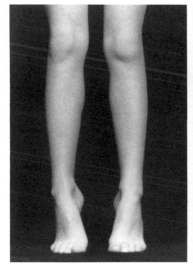
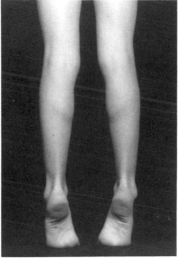

The next stage is to move the feet apart.

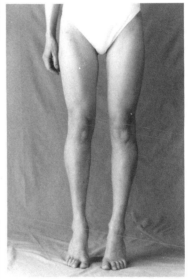

Mistakes tend to increase as the contact between the malleoli is lost. Have a partner guide you, or work in front of a full-length mirror. As always, the patella should be positioned above the second toe. In the mirror, the heel should not stick out to the right or left.

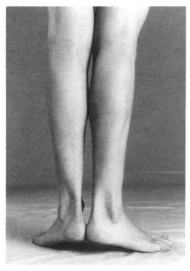
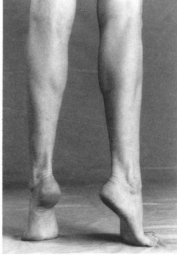

Add lateral rotation of the hips. Maintain the weight on the toes, patellas above the second toes, and feeling of muscular tightening in the leg.

Be conscious of the position of the heels. As you begin to stand on the toes, the heels should be close together. They move away from each other only near maximum height. Similarly, when coming down, the heels move together again before they reach the floor.

As your technique improves, try standing on the toes of one foot. This is good preparation for many spins and jumps. Finally, try all these variations without holding on to any support.

Softening the impact in jumps*

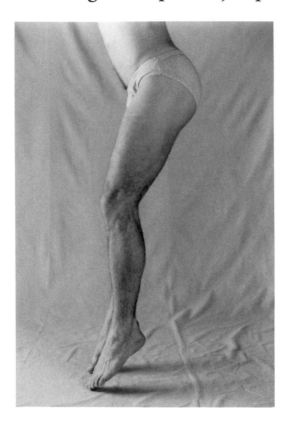

In French, the word "amortissement" is often used to refer to a non-traumatic landing from a jump.

It is defined as "reducing the effect." Depending on our technique, landing from a jump can be jarring or barely felt.

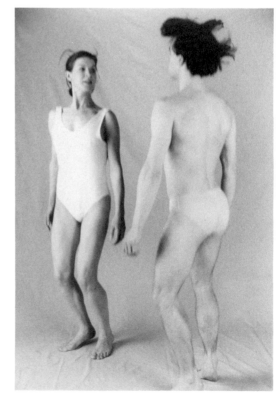

Three factors help soften the landing phase of a jump:

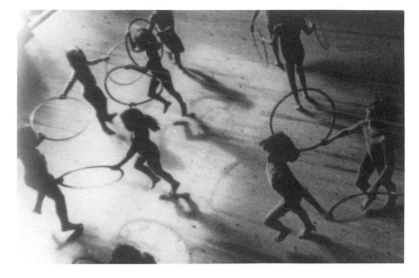

- The floor itself. Concrete, tile over concrete, or wood over concrete will always provide a hard, unyielding surface. Wood floors supported by beams, but with much empty space under them, provide a softer, more yielding landing surface. The ideal exercise room has this type of floor.

- Shoes with soles designed to cushion impact, such as the many styles of "walking" and "cross-training" shoes popular today. We insist on the use of such shoes when exercising on hard floors. Likewise, a bulky sweater tied around the waist helps protect the pelvic bones in exercise situations where falls are frequent.

- Through appropriate movements and adjustments, the body itself can act as an "amortisseur," or "device used in cushioning the impact of a violent shock." This is our focus in this section.

Learning to land softly benefits you in both a short-term and a long-term sense. To understand why, think about what happens when shocks are not cushioned properly. Consider a hypothetical dancer who jumps bare-footed onto a concrete floor for 30 minutes without making any attempt to soften the landing impact. Every time he hits the floor the impact is transmitted from the feet all the way to the skull through a series of bones and joints. It is like hitting all these structures repeatedly with a hammer.

Think about the cartilage which covers the articulating ends of bones (see *AOM*, p. 11). One of its main functions is to act as a shock absorber. Over the course of time, if stresses are too intense or too often repeated, cartilage can become thin, cracked, or worn out. Remember that cartilage has no blood supply of its own. It depends on the proximity of synovial fluid, or capillaries of the perichondrium or periosteum, for delivery of nutrients or removal of waste products. Therefore, when a cartilage is injured, healing is very slow or may not occur at all. Cartilages are fragile tissues which must be protected as much as possible in our daily activities as well as during vigorous exercise. Deterioration, inflammation, and loss of mobility in joint cartilage (arthrosis or arthritis) cause pain and stiffening, and may even incapacitate us.

Impact-softening techniques should be taught at the earliest stages of physical disciplines.

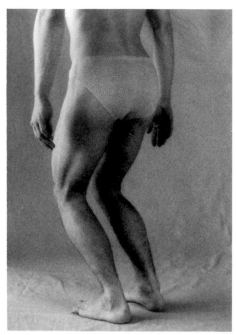

We will describe an effective way to soften landing impact from a straight vertical jump, where the feet are parallel and hip-width apart. Work on this technique until it becomes "automatic."

It can then be extended to more complex jumps, such as:

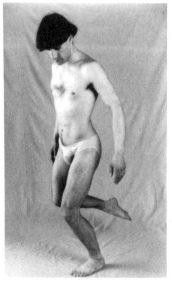

• one legged

• with forward or lateral propulsion, or turning

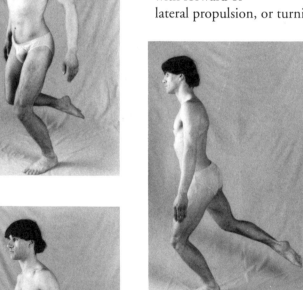

• with lateral rotation of the hips (in ballet or some martial arts)

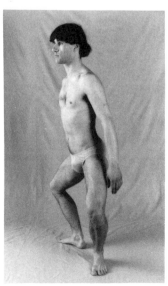

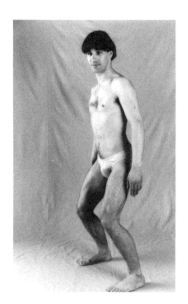

• with the legs greater distances apart

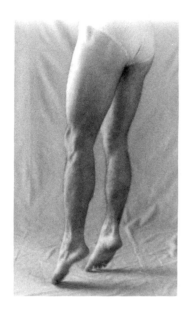

A slow-motion description of the ideal landing is as follows. Start with the body at the apex of the jump, in mid-air. As contact is made with the ground, there is a smooth, continuous "rolling" movement along the foot in the sequence:

- tips of the big toes

- bottoms of all toes

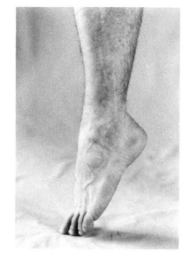

- metatarsal heads

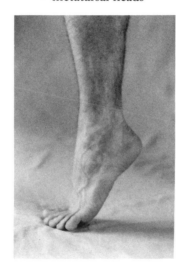

- arches

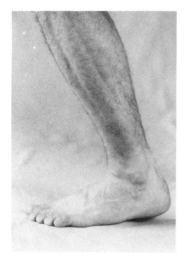

- heel

This sequence is synchronized with progressive and simultaneous flexion of the ankles, knees, and hips.

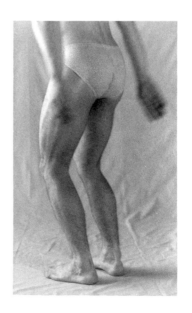

The trunk should remain essentially vertical and straight on the flexed lower limbs, and located above the heels, as in the plié.

What are the common obstacles to this idealized, synchronized movement?

- Restricted ROM somewhere along the line. The "rolling" will stop at the restricted area.

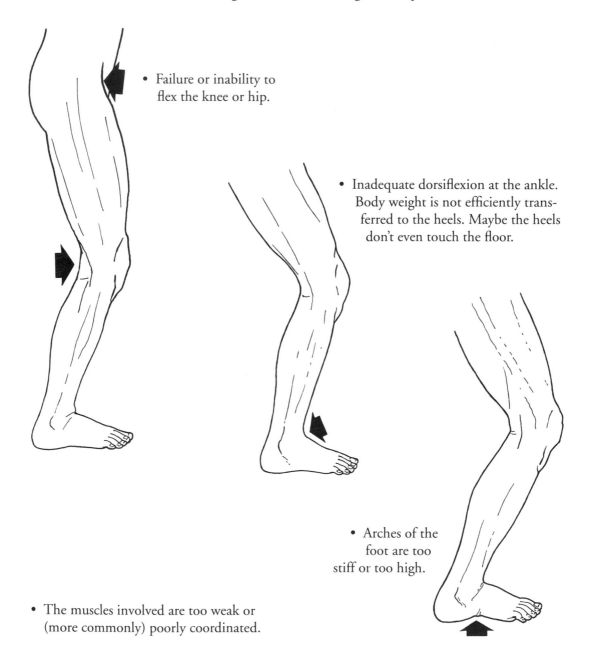

- Failure or inability to flex the knee or hip.

- Inadequate dorsiflexion at the ankle. Body weight is not efficiently transferred to the heels. Maybe the heels don't even touch the floor.

- Arches of the foot are too stiff or too high.

- The muscles involved are too weak or (more commonly) poorly coordinated.

How can you recognize an uncushioned landing impact?
- You hear a loud noise of impact as the feet hit the floor.
- The heels do not touch the floor.
- Visually, you get an impression of stiffness or lack of coordination.

To improve articular ROMs, spend some time on the limbering exercises described in previous chapters for the hip (see p. 160), knee (p. 196), and ankle (p. 224).

Next, we will link together two basic exercises described earlier in this chapter:

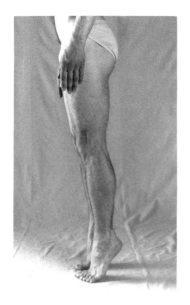

- Standing on the toes (see p. 258),

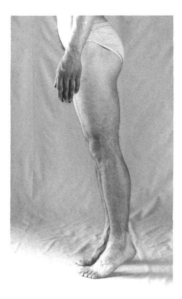

coming down,

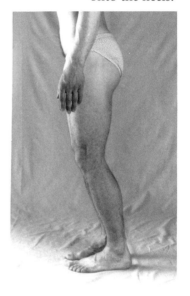

shifting the body weight onto the heels.

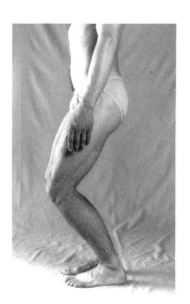

- Half plié (see pp. 252–253). With the medial malleoli together, lower the trunk as much as possible while still keeping the heels on the floor, as if sitting straight down onto them.

How do we link these two movements together? Start with a preparatory exercise: stand up with legs straight. Shift the body weight forward, then backward, then again forward in a flowing action. Next, from a position with body weight on the toes and metatarsal heads, lower the feet back down flat (body weight on the heels) and link this to the half plié where the heels stay on the floor.

To improve the transition from the up to the down position, you need to learn how to flex the knees just before the heels reach the floor. This creates a more "flowing" movement and is the key to a soft, quiet landing. Here is a useful exercise:

Without lifting the toes off the floor, raise and lower the heels only.

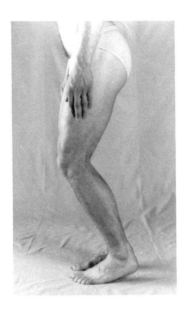 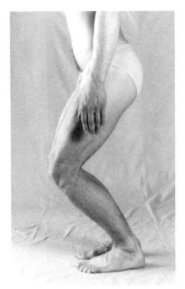

Gradually increase the speed of this movement. Think about a flowing movement of flexion at the knee and ankle. Your goal at this stage is to improve coordination of everything that happens up to the knee.

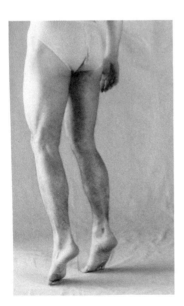 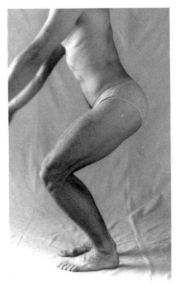

You may need to temporarily "accept the mistake" of the buttocks sticking out too much, because this helps maintain balance at the landing phase of a jump, when flexibility is still not sufficient at the ankles. In other words, as long as the ankles are not ready (this may take several months), allow the trunk to lean forward.

Proper cushioning of landing impact is a technique which, once well-practiced and understood, stays with you no matter what difficulties are added later as you learn more complex jumps. Conversely, people who have grown accustomed to landing in an incorrect manner have a hard time "unlearning" the bad technique. The simplest criterion is: a good landing is a quiet landing.

Softening the impact in walking*

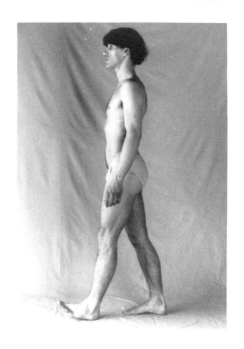

The landing phase in jumping is essentially vertical. In walking, by contrast, the body and feet are moving primarily in a horizontal direction. The heel, not the toe, is the first part of the foot to contact the floor. There is no need for the rolling movement of the foot, nor the simultaneous flexion of the ankle, knee and hip, as described above for jumping.

Some people hit the floor too hard with the heel during normal walking. On hardwood floors, this produces a characteristic loud thumping noise. Visually, this way of walking gives an impression of heaviness, especially when walking down stairs. It is often associated with a forward-leaning body posture (see pp. 222–23).

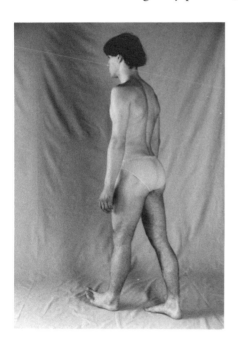

Why is this? When the body habitually leans forward during walking, the body's weight always "wants" to shift immediately to the front of the foot at each step, and the heel hits the floor abruptly and heavily. This repeated impact to the heel is transmitted straight up through the leg bones and spine, and can eventually damage the cartilages of the knees or even the vertebrae.

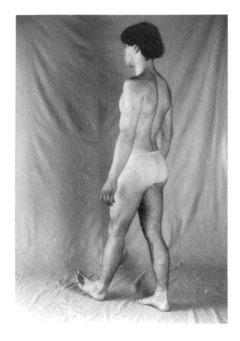

When the body is held more to the back, its weight is not transferred immediately to the front foot at each step, and there is a more gradual shift of weight from the heel to the front. The heel does not hit so heavily, and there is less noise.

Thus, softening the impact during walking depends less on actions of the leg than on where the body's center of gravity is carried.

Propulsion in walking

The word "propulsion" comes from the Latin "propellere": to push forward. Our interest is in forward, horizontal propulsion in walking and running, and vertical propulsion in jumping.

In walking, there are two different means of forward propulsion. In one, the head and shoulders are held forward, the body's center of gravity is over the front foot, there is a general loss of balance toward the front, and the legs must move to recover balance.

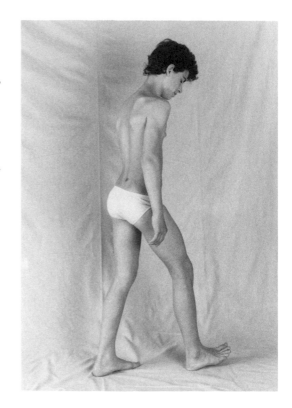

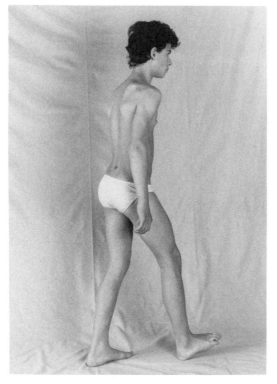

Essentially, the feet are following the trunk. This type of walking doesn't require much muscular work by the legs, particularly by the gluteals or the ankle dorsiflexors. On the other hand, the posterior trunk muscles must stay contracted to support the forward-leaning position.

In the second type of walking, the body's center of gravity is more vertical. The legs must move the trunk rather than vice versa. The propulsion comes from pushing of the feet against the floor rather than falling forward of the torso. In analyzing this type of walking, we should look at four different regions and their movements.

1. Plantar flexion of foot

The foot pushes off the floor in a sequential manner, with the area of propulsion moving from back to front:

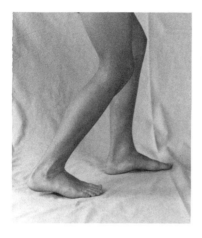

- The heel lifts, and weight is on the lateral arch. Active muscles: gastrocnemius, soleus.

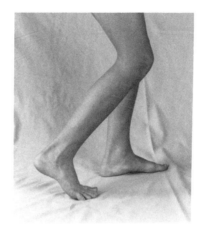

- The midfoot lifts, and weight is on the metatarsal heads. Active muscles: peroneus longus, tibialis posterior.

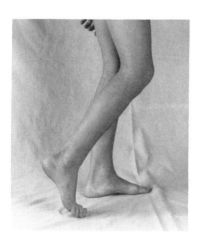

- The metatarsal heads lift, and then the toes in sequence. Active muscles: flexor digitorum longus, other toe flexors.

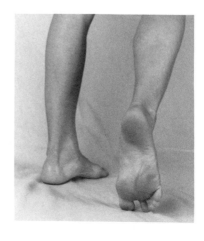

- The big toe gives a last push as the foot completely leaves the floor. Active muscle: flexor hallucis longus. When we wear shoes, this action is prevented, which is unfortunate because this muscle is essential for the stability of the ankle and foot (see p. 240), and this is a good exercise for it.

2. Extension of hip

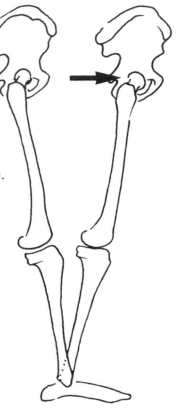

In some cases, ROM for this movement
may be deficient. To regain extension ROM,
see the sections on hip flexibility (p. 162)
and horizontal movements of the pelvis (p. 178).

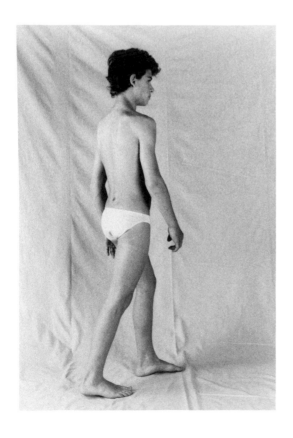

It may also be necessary to "activate"
gluteus maximus, the main hip extensor.
When walking, try keeping the body
weight on the heel as long as possible,
and visualize the anterior horizontal
movement of the pelvis (p. 178).
Don't confuse this with lordosis
of the lumbar spine.

3. Extension of knee

This occurs at a certain stage of walking propulsion. ROM for knee extension can be improved by the following exercise. Stand with one leg back and the other forward. Keep the body weight on the back foot, and slightly bend that knee. Keeping the pelvis fixed, try to simultaneously extend the back of the knee (popliteal fossa) and the front of the hip.

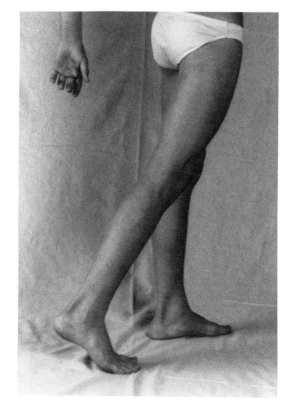

There are two muscular actions going on here. The hip extension activates the rectus femoris which, when stretched, tends to extend the knee. The knee extension activates the hamstrings, which in turn, when stretched, tend to tilt the pelvis in retroversion (which facilitates hip extension). Thus, there is a reciprocal facilitation of the rectus femoris and hamstrings, and this completes the action of the gluteus maximus.

4. Dorsiflexion of ankle

The exercise described above is enhanced by pressing the heel against the floor (ankle dorsiflexion), which stretches the two heads of gastrocnemius. When the foot is not bearing weight, gastrocnemius flexes the knee. However, when the two heads are stretched by ankle dorsiflexion, they pull the femoral condyles posteriorly and take the knee into extension. This reinforces the hip extension/knee extension positive feedback loop described above.

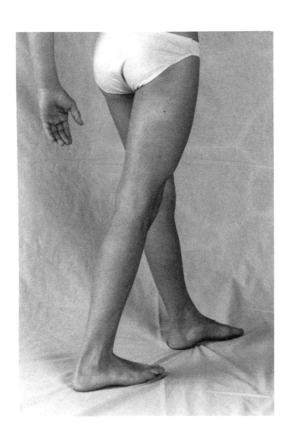

Keep the heel pressed down as long as possible before returning to phase one of the propulsion cycle, in which the foot pushes off again. Combine this propulsion sequence with "guiding of the leg from the foot" (see p. 250). By walking this way, you involve all the muscles of the thigh and leg.

Propulsion in running

In walking, there is always at least one foot (and often both) in contact with the ground. In running, the two feet are never on the ground simultaneously, and there are appreciable periods when neither foot is touching the ground. The force of propulsion must be more powerful than in walking. Much of the force is provided by the bulkiest muscles: quadriceps femoris (extending the knee) and gastrocnemius (plantar flexing the ankle). The upper body (and consequently the center of gravity) are shifted forward and off balance, and the legs are always working to keep up. Thus, the weight is always on the anterior foot, and phase four as described for walking (where the heel pushes against the ground) cannot occur.

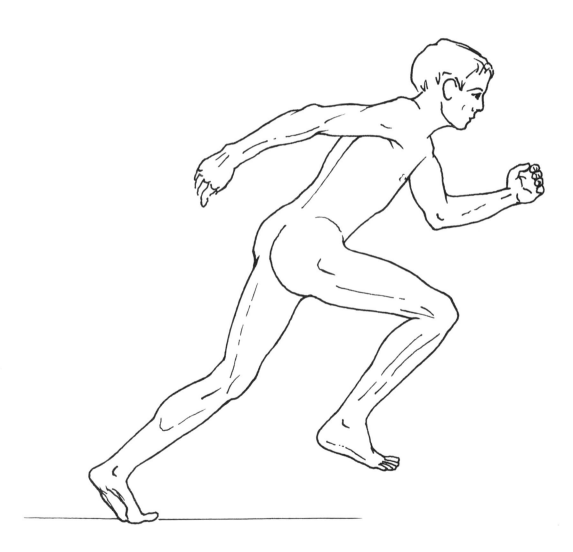

Propulsion in jumping

Vertical jumping

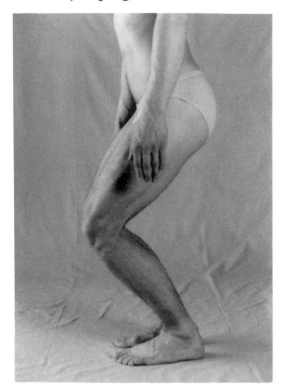

This involves a transition from "triple flexion" (dorsiflexion of ankle, flexion of knee and hip) . . .

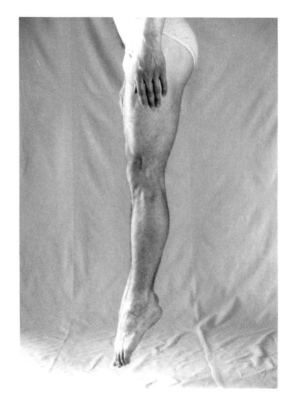

. . . to "triple extension" (plantar flexion of ankle, extension of knee and hip).

This is the reverse of landing from a jump (see p. 263). The muscles which are the prime movers in vertical jumping act as brakes in landing from a jump.

High jumping requires good articular ROM, muscular strength, and speed of muscle contraction. Speed will be enhanced by prior stretching of the muscles, i.e., you need to start low to jump high.

Jumping forward

This involves a combination of the propulsion factors for walking and vertical jumping.

Index

....

T